HEAL &
PREVENT
STROKE & HEART DISEASE

HEAL &
PREVENT
STROKE & HEART DISEASE

PREM K. BHANDARI

iUniverse, Inc.

New York Bloomington Shanghai

Heal & Prevent Stroke & Heart Disease

iUniverse books may be ordered through booksellers or by contacting:

iUniverse
1663 Liberty Drive
Bloomington, IN 47403
www.iuniverse.com
1-800-Authors (1-800-288-4677)

Because of the dynamic nature of the Internet, any Web addresses or links contained in this book may have changed since publication and may no longer be valid.

The information, ideas, and suggestions in this book are not intended as a substitute for professional medical advice. Before following any suggestions contained in this book, you should consult your personal physician. Neither the author nor the publisher shall be liable or responsible for any loss or damage allegedly arising as a consequence of your use or application of any information or suggestions in this book.

ISBN: 978-0-595-41870-1 (pbk)
ISBN: 978-0-595-86217-7 (ebk)

Printed in the United States of America

CONTENTS

CHAPTER I

INTRODUCTION

For several years, I thought about writing a book on my experiences of living and working in various parts of the world. But each time I started to write, something more urgent and crucially important to my livelihood pulled me in another direction. I was in good health and enjoyed an active, athletic, and joyful life. I had successfully overcome minor health problems before, and believed that nothing serious could go wrong with my health. This gave me the confidence that I would be able to overcome any health problem should it ever surface. Also, I never realized that I was getting old like every body else, and my confidence in maintaining good health indefinitely under a stressful business environment could be suddenly shattered. It did get shattered in 1996 and 1997 when I suffered from series of strokes and angina attacks. I had been a fitness conscious sportsman, very aware of what it took to maintain all aspects of my health, and was totally unprepared for what lay ahead. After the stroke and angina attacks, I could not walk up and down stairs. I could not remember the names of my relatives. I could not speak, read, and understand others. My vision was at minimum. I could not even remember if I had enough money in the bank to support myself to the end of the month. My memory was lost.

But I did recover. I learned to heal myself from the aftermath of strokes and angina attacks, and I relearned everything I know today through my own efforts. As I did, I developed a system for recovering from stoke and heart attack that I am now sharing with you. I feel fortunate to restore my lost vision, speech fluency, memory, and various physical functions. I did it without any medication. In the process, I received a good lesson from the healthcare industry—that our health system is commerce based, and the patient must take control of managing his or her own recovery.

I want to be able to help as many people as I can to learn to deal with stroke and heart disease, recover from such conditions, and not experience them again. Also, this book may generate some income for my senior years which have already arrived. In this book I have briefly described my own experiences with cardio vascular disease, and made an attempt to demonstrate ways to self manage such conditions in a simple and easy to understand language.

The healthcare industry is a provider of healthcare services to the population—it is a business—like any other service provider. Healthcare is only one of several important aspects of our life, and the industry should not be allowed to take the patient from one stage to another. No doubt, the healthcare industry can prove to be the most important service to the population under abnormal health conditions; however, they should not be allowed to take a patient from one stage to another under normal health conditions.

The human body is imperfect, and if we play with it too much then we dig up just about every ailment there can be. Already people are getting treated for the ailments that have not even surfaced yet. People are taking medication in doses that are not necessary. Children are on medication. It seems that we want to cure every ailment, and kill every germ that exists, which is quite impractical. Industries within the commercial environment do produce innovation through continuous research and development under a competitive environment, but when such industries happen to be in the arena of human well being, and then the equation becomes somewhat different. Inherent contradiction exists between the need for the medical industry to make profits, and the need for the population to receive much needed healthcare in the most unbiased manner. Why would the medical professionals and the hospitals not exploit such a lucrative business option? After all they did not put up their shops for humanitarian reasons; they are in business to make money, and money they make. No matter how many laws may be regulating them, they will make money one way or another, which should be acceptable to all of us because they do provide a tremendous contribution to the society, and have successfully demonstrated this by lengthening the average life span.

Does it pay to be a patient unless it is a life threatening emergency? During life threatening emergencies the healthcare community makes the most money. Do they invite such emergencies to knock on their doors? Of course not. Humans create the conditions through their lifestyles that demand medical services in the marketplace, that is, besides the physiological slow down due to the aging process.

I suggest that under the business environment, each patient should act like a business person, and should take control of the management of his or her health. The majority of people, including myself, never dare to ask doctors any questions, or if the question is asked, we tend to agree before they even complete their response. We become agreeable when we face a healthcare professional. This is our training which demands that healthcare professionals should be given utmost respect and their word be the final word. I was taught to carry the thought that all medical professionals mean well. I would like to see every patient or non-patient manage their own health affairs, and make a lot of related conversations with the healthcare professionals regarding anything and everything connected with patient's health condition and the cure. This method will reduce the public dependency on the over burdened healthcare system, people would try to stay healthier, healthcare costs will be reduced, and the healthcare professionals will have more time to focus on patients who require more attention. Also, this will keep the healthcare professionals on their toes, which will make them more alert. On the flip side, this will discourage patients who just happen to be in the habit of rushing to the clinic for extremely minor ailments, which could be looked after by them at home, or could be discussed with the nurse over the telephone. The pharmacists at the drugstores are very knowledgeable and they are fully capable of advising patients about most minor health conditions, which relate to over the counter drugs. After all, they fill a large number of prescriptions each day, which happens to keep them in business.

This book is not meant to reduce the importance of the healthcare providers and professionals, but is for raising the awareness of the general population and especially the stroke and heart patients who can play a much more active role in the management of their health, and the healing process of their health condition. They do not need to leave everything to the medical professionals to heal them and keep them healthy. Hopefully, I will motivate many patients to recover more speedily than it would happen otherwise. This book is also directed to those who want to prevent cardio vascular disease and the occurrences related to it. It is better to be proactive especially in respect to health, and being in charge is very important and simple.

I am a self taught person who has been interested in science from childhood. This interest in science prompted me to read many authors on diversified scientific disciplines. In this book, I have provided various data only to draw attention to the severity of the impact of cardiovascular disease in the United States. Also, I have provided various brief explanations about stroke and heart disease; you will see that the causes of this disease are just a few and they are curable.

This book goes through the healing process step by step. I have given a brief description of my experiences and the methods I developed and practiced to heal my condition without medication. A brief description of some of the specific therapies and exercises are provided; they are strictly the outcome of my own training as I was growing up, as well as my own methods developed through trial and error. All these diets and therapies worked for me in restoring my memory, communications, vision, muscles, stamina, energy, balance, coordination, and comprehension. My system enabled me to participate in life again.

In this book I share my experience of learning with others so that they too can benefit. If I could do it without any medical help, medicine, and caregiver, then you can most certainly do it too. However, do take advantage of the medical help if you have it, but remain a manager of your own health.

I would like the readers of this book to notice the fact that I am not a physician, medical researcher or professional in any scientific discipline, and I am not attempting to confirm the accuracy, promote, or market any of the statistical and technical data in this book. Also, I am not affiliated with any group, industry, association, or business in the medical, healthcare, food, and nutritional supplement industry. During a period of 5 decades, I read many books, journals, research materials, and reference books related to various sciences which include physiology, biology, healthcare, nutrition, diseases, and various other related scientific disciplines. I continue to do so. Most of the statistical and technical data mentioned in this book have been selected and derived from numerous sources that are freely available in the public libraries, reference books, periodicals, US Government publications, AHA, CDC, NIH, ASA, DHHS, USDA, FDA, and many other sources on the internet. Choice of foods, therapies, learning processes, preventions, safeguards, and attitudes have been developed by me through my own trial and error methods based on the day to day conditions as a stroke patient, state of mind, upbringing, and witnessing the effects of heart disease in my family since very young age.

Having been born and raised in New Delhi, India I was exposed to foods that are now classified as alternative foods, exercises, philosophy, therapies, and lifestyle at an early age. This lifestyle, which is thousands of years old, is second nature to me. These alternatives are ingrained in me and I am thankful for it. In many cases, this knowledge enables me to go beyond the current practices of the medical community. The statistical data and technical explanations have been introduced only to underscore the importance of having a proper lifestyle that is conducive to healing and prevention for the stroke and heart disease patients and potential patients. Also, this book contains my opinions, beliefs, and perceptions based on my heritage, experience, and health condition.

I feel fortunate to have read several books on the related subjects and was able to determine the common theme of various health conditions and the relative chain of causes thereof. Some of these writers are: A. P. Fishman, D. W. Richards, Ruth Singer, Zsolt Harsanyi, Richard Hutton, Earle Hackett, Alexander Grant, Andrew Weil, Ross Trattler, Carlson Wade, Robert Becker, Gary Selden, Floyd Chilton, Laura Tucker, Joseph Mercola, J. D. Decuypere, Wanda Hamilton, Nir Barzilai, Claudia Dreifus, Richard Senelick, Karla Dougherty, lawrence Agress; Cotran, Kumar, Robbins, M. Aviram & K. Eias, R. A. Karmali, J. M. Kremer, H. R. Knapp, Paul Schulick, J. E. Brody, Robert Becker, A. Cassidy, Joseph Wepman, Carlson Wade, Laurie Deutsch Mozian, David Weibers, Michael Mogadam, Time Life publications, Newsweek, Better Homes & Garden, various scientific publications in the UK, USA, India, Singapore, Thailand, Canada and France, various Medical Dictionaries and Encyclopedias, various science journals & periodicals, conversations with professionals in various parts of the world, and attending health related events. I am also grateful to the writers and scholars whose names I do not remember but from whom I learned a lot. It will be impossible for me to quote all sources of reading and learning about various related sciences during the past 50-plus years. The contents of this book are strictly for information and knowledge purposes, and before putting any of the contents to practice the reader should consult his or her personal physician.

CHAPTER II

SCOPE & SYMPTOMS OF STROKE & HEART DISEASE

Historically, people have associated stroke and heart condition with males only, probably because most of the time males complained, and got attended to. The ones who knew something about it had little or no knowledge about its causes, let alone its cure. Females were never considered as candidates for such health conditions, even though they experienced a variety of stress levels; in many cases even higher than males. Somehow for unspecified reasons, the medical community ignored them. **Unattended stroke and heart patients can die slowly, and women did die of stroke and heart attacks over thousands of years without being attended to.** The cause of their death remained unknown, or kept confidential for cultural or religious reasons, or labeled as female disease. It is beyond the comprehension of most people that women who gave birth and life to us, raised us, and cared for all of us at every micro step of the way to adulthood, and provided so much care to all of us humans even after we were able to take care of ourselves, were not only denied but ignored for the essential basics of healthcare under stroke and heart condition. Just visualize the degree of agony and sorrow these female stroke and heart patients must have experienced. Healthcare should be available to all human beings, no matter how minimal it may be, with a special emphasis of attention to women whose importance and major role in everyone's life cannot be ignored. It is cynical of humanity to degrade about half of it (female population) which provides life, birth, care, and undulating love to all of us, by ignoring them when they are in need of medical help under stroke or heart condition.

According to Center for Disease Control, cardio vascular disease (CVD) causes more than 900,000 deaths each year in the USA, which includes heart attack, stroke, and related deaths. If all the artery diseases are included with CVD, the number of deaths each year in the USA climbs up to a several million. All research analysis had been broken down to several layers of CVD, which is one way to identify the proximate cause of the disease and to cure it. Also, we cannot ignore the fact that proportionately women suffer from Cardio Vascular Disease as much as men do, that is, when women are fortunate to get diagnosed and medically cared for. It is estimated that about 61% of all CVD related deaths were women.

American Heart & Stroke Association indicates that about 1.2 million Americans, suffer from coronary heart disease, both first time and repeated, each year. Each year, about 13.2 million Americans experience the occurrence of Angina and Coronary Heart Disease. Out of these numbers, 7.2 million among the males, and 6 million among females suffer from this. About half a million die from it each year. What a pity.

Stroke kills a little over 162.000 Americans each year, and at least 50% of them happen to be women. 2.4 million Men and 3 million women suffer from Stroke each year. There are 500,000 new cases of stroke each year in addition to 200,000 recurrent cases each year. Also there are estimated 5.5 million stroke survivors live today.

Cardio Vascular Disease encompasses a select group of diseases that are immediately related to heart and stroke conditions. There are about 71 million Americans who suffer from cardio vascular disease. Out of this number about 13.2 million is credited to Coronary Heart Disease, 7.2 million suffer from Acute Heart Attack or Myocardial Infarction. About 6.5 million Americans experience Angina each year. Angina is acute discomfort caused by blockage of blood supply to the heart. Exact number of deaths from Angina is not known, but it is a staggering one.

In 2002, a study showed that Stroke killed 162,672 people. Ironically, 61% of them were women. These numbers demonstrate how little attention women have received over the years. Women were considered second class citizens. Black women have experienced much more disadvantage over white women. In 2002, per 100,000 people in the USA,

   82 black and 54 white men
   72 black and 53 white women
   48 men and women from Asian origin
   41 men and women from the Latino group
   37 men and women of American Indian & Alaska natives
died from the Stroke. 50% of Stroke Deaths occur before the person reaches hospital. So the recognition of stroke symptoms is absolutely important and crucial. Earlier the symptoms are recognized the faster will be the arrival of the patient at the hospital for the treatment.

American Heart Association has developed a consolidated data for 2003 on Cardio Vascular disease, and according to them total CVD related deaths in 2003 were 1.4 million. In other words, one out of every 2.7 deaths, approximately, occurred in the USA was due to cardio vascular disease. Deaths resulting from various conditions of cardio vascular disease have been further broken down as: 53% died of coronary heart disease, 17% died of stroke, 6% died of heart failure, 6% died of high blood pressure, 4% died of arterial disease, 04% died of rheumatic heart disease, 0.5% died of congenital cardio vascular defects, etc. In 2003 about 6.8 million in-patients were subjected to cardio vascular related operations, 2003 statistics also indicates that 50% of men and 89% of women who died suddenly due to coronary heart disease had no prior history, nor any symptoms whatsoever. Additionally, people who have suffered a heart attack before, have a sudden death rate that is 4 to 6 times higher than that of the rest of the population. Stroke ranks # 3 after heart and cancer related deaths. Every 3 minutes someone dies of stroke. These statistics are scary and require attention.

Each year, about 700,000 men and women suffer a Stroke out of which 500,000 are the first timers, and 200,000 are second or third or fourth. Each year Medicare spends billions of dollars on Stroke Survivors after they leave hospitals. Now, who can question the importance of stroke or heart attack incidence in the USA, and its subsequent impact on the survivors and the loved ones? If you experience stroke or heart attack once, then that should be more than enough; you do not need the second one, or even third one. The best thing is to avoid the first occurrence of stroke or heart attack, and the second best is never let it happen again. How to avoid stroke or heart attack in the first place is not difficult at all, if one knows about it and how to read in to the symptoms. Anyone can prevent stroke or heart attack occurrence.

Quite often thoughts come in to my mind and in millions of others, regarding the miseries, upheavals, stress, health problems, etc. each of us experience during our life time. Individually, we think it is happening to us only, but the truth is such unwanted things are being experienced by every one of us on this planet, in one way or another. Are we pre-ordained for our experiences? Not really. If there was no food, then humans would be eating vegetation to survive, and if there was no medical help then humans will do whatever it takes to stay alive and healthy. Of course, not too many would survive without medical help if a major disease came upon us. But most of us would try our best to survive, because we all have been genetically endowed with the instinct to survive. Most certainly, we do not have to abandon this instinct to survive under modern conditions where a significant amount of medical help is available and can be sought. This is the very instinct that helps most people to survive under unbearable and adverse conditions. Why can't we use this natural gift of survival under modern conditions when abundant food supply and medical help are available? In spite of this affluence, people still die. In fact, medical help cannot guarantee, beyond a certain limit, life, longevity, or good health to any one on this planet, whether it happens to be a human or any other species of animal kingdom, without the will and active participation of the subject. We should never succumb to the thought that if medical help did not arrive, or was not available for one reason or another, it is the end of the world. Without our individual desire and will to survive, even the best medical help cannot help us. It is within us that instigate the survival process, and it has never existed outside of our mind. Please do remember this important attribute, because this is the only thing that will help you survive a stroke, heart attack, or any other serious health condition, no matter how sophisticated medical help you may receive during a very trying period of serious health crisis.

Medical community and research institutes are becoming aware of the fact that medicines help to guard the body temporarily, and only to boost the system temporarily, and once the immune system is good and running the body cures the health problem itself. Medicines help, to boost the immune system, but do not cure the ailment in most cases. Here, the patients' 'will' to get healed, and his or her active participation become of prime importance. Surgery is a great trauma to the body, but in the same manner our immune system takes over and heals it. The healing process of the body is tied to our immune system, our instinct to survive, our attitude, and our active participation to get healed. They are all interrelated and not separated.

Knowledge of CVD (cardio vascular disease) symptoms could bring you closer to recovery; however, ignorance could bring you closer to death or disability. Learn about your own body's responses to various ailments, stroke and heart conditions, and various circumstances of your own life. Most definitely, each human being is entirely different from the other. There are probably billions and billions of variable combinations that are unique to each human in the way of habits, likes, dislikes, personality profile, emotions, life style, life circumstances, relative and specific responses to each event, etc., and therefore knowing yourself is of immense importance in enjoying a healthy life and avoiding a stroke or heart attack occurrence. Medical help comes in a form of a blanket which would fit all. If the individual knows what to do in a certain situation, that individual will be able to tackle the situation much better than the one who does not know. Knowledge of stroke or heart condition and its related issues would greatly help any one to avoid stroke or heart attack occurrence.

When blood supply in a part of brain is interrupted by blockage of blood vessel or a rupture of blood vessel, thereby allowing the blood to flow in to brain tissue and resulting in the injury or complete destruction of brain neurons in an area of brain then it is called an incidence of "stroke". If the blood supply to the brain is disrupted, brain cells can die or get damaged. This condition is identified as "stroke". Stroke is a brain injury caused by death or damage of brain cells and/or neurons. Neurons are responsible for sending messages to all parts of the body, and therefore control just about every function of the body.

Stroke used to be known as "Apoplexy" which is a Greek word meaning strike down, which is quite literal and appropriate for the incidence of stroke. Stroke is also known as "Cerebral-vascular Accident". Stroke is Brain Attack which occurs in the brain just like Heart Attack which occurs in the heart.

Stroke or Brain Attack is third largest cause of death, and it is the leading cause of disability in the United States. When stroke happens to be in the left side of the brain, then the right side of the body is adversely affected by paralysis, numbness, inability to function properly, complete disability in some physical functions restrictive movement, insensitivity in some areas, etc. speech, spoken and written language understanding difficulties, etc., etc.

When stroke happens to be in the right side of the brain, then the left side of the body is adversely affected, vision is blurred and out of focus, perception and dimensions become unreal, etc. Overall, language, communications abilities, memory, paralysis, etc. are the outcomes of a stroke incidence. Even personality can be altered by a stroke.

Medical community has classified strokes which happen to be of various types. New names would emerge as medical researchers discover new types in the future. Some of these types of strokes have been briefly introduced here.

ISCHEMIC STROKE:

It is a common knowledge that blood clotting is beneficial especially when we are bleeding from a wound. Blood clots work to stop, or at least slow the bleeding, and thereby creating a condition for the wound to heal. Blood clots are dangerous for the body, because they can block arteries and cut off the flow of blood, which leads to stroke conditions that can be fatal. There is Transient Ischemic Attack (TIA) which is stroke like attack, and is called the first warning sign of an oncoming Brain Attack or Stroke in the future. An Ischemic attack can occur in another way.: The other way is when the blockage occurs in the coronary artery which supplies blood and oxygen to the heart, and this condition is known as heart disease which can lead to heart attack.

EMBOLIC STROKE

When a blood clot originating from somewhere in the body (quite often from the heart), and then travels through to the brain, and enters into a small blood vessel (tube) and blocks it.

Ischemic Stroke is the most common type of stroke experienced by people

20% mortality within 30 days

60% survive the first year, and 50% in 5 year period

60%–70% of survivors suffer some disability immediately after the stroke

40% in 6 months, and 30% in one year

THROMBOTIC STROKE

When the blood clot forms within the blood vessel locally, thereby blocking it; this occurrence is called Thrombosis Stroke it is caused by built up of fatty deposits and Cholesterol. They cause multiple levels of tiny and multiple injuries to the blood vessel walls. The incidence of these injuries gets repeated regularly. Our bodies react to these injuries and tend to repair them. Just like if we are bleeding from a wound our bodies respond by forming blood clots to stop bleeding, similarly our bodies form blood clots to repair these injuries, or stop bleeding if some bleeding occurs inside these injured blood vessels. There are two types of Thrombosis that can cause Stroke: Large Vessel Thrombosis, and Small Vessel Disease

LARGE VESSEL THROMBOSIS

It occurs in the large arteries, and is the best understood one. Most of the time, it is caused by sustained and long term Arteriosclerosis which promotes rapid blood clot formation by the body. Large Vessel Thrombosis does not show immediate symptoms of injuries to the walls and therefore remain unnoticed for some time during which body continuously forms clots to conduct repairs. And one or more clots end up blocking blood vessels in the brain, thereby causing stroke (brain attack).

Thrombosis Stroke patients are most likely to have the disease of Coronary Artery, and Heart Attack is a common cause of death in patients who have suffered this kind of Brain Attack or Stroke.

SMALL VESSEL DISEASE

Small Vessel Disease, also known as Lacunars Infarction, occurs when blood flow is blocked to very small arteries. It is closely linked to hypertension which is caused by high blood pressure. Very little is known about this disease, and like any other related disease, it is under extensive research.

HEMORRHAGE STROKE

Hemorrhage stroke can be defined as the breakage or blow out of a blood vessel in the brain, and is caused by High blood pressure, and Cerebral Aneurysm. We already know what high blood pressure is. Aneurysm is a thin or weak spot on a blood vessel. These weak spots are present at birth, and do not pose any detectable problems until they break. There are two types of Hemorrhagic Strokes.

SUB-ARACHNOID HEMORRHAGE (SAH)

An Aneurism bursts in a large artery on the thin and delicate membrane, or around it that surrounds the brain. As a result of this burst, blood oozes out and spills in to the area around the brain. There is a fluid that surrounds and protects the brain. The spilled blood gets mixed with this protective liquid and contaminates it

SYMPTOMS OF SUB ARACHNOID HEMORRHAGE (SAH)

- Very severe headache, kind of worst headache
- Intolerance to light and brightness
- Stiff neck area
- Feeling of vomiting and nausea
- Loss of consciousness
- Partial loss of vision, speech, understanding, reading and writing etc.
- Partial memory loss
- Vision impairment
- Off-balance, confusion, dizziness, helplessness, feeling of insecurity

  Sub Arachinoid Hemorrhage has
  40% mortality within 30 days of experiencing stroke
  50% of the survivors have disability.

INTRA-CEREBRAL HEMORRHAGE (ICH)

Intra-Cerebral Hemorrhage is when bleeding occurs within a blood vessel in the brain itself. High blood pressure and hypertension are the primary causes of this Brain Attack, or Stroke. It is a major type of stroke.

SYMPTOMS OF INTRA-CEREBRAL HEMORRHAGE (ICH)

Symptoms may vary depending upon the specific location and the amount of bleeding in the brain. However, major symptoms are:

- Excruciating and severe headache like not having experienced before
- Sudden weakness felt in the legs, joints, arms, face,
- Feeling of nausea, vomiting,
- Partial or total loss of consciousness

- Balance and coordination
- Walking difficulties, dizziness
- Partial memory loss

Regular and smooth flow of blood supply to the brain is crucial to its function. Blood rich in oxygen and other nutrients to feed the brain 24 hours a day via sophisticated system of blood carrying vessels is absolutely essential for the brain to function and stay alive. Brain is

2% of an adult's body weight

It receives about

20% of body's oxygen

15% of heart's output of fresh blood

100% of liver's output of glucose or blood sugar

Brain has no storage facility, and therefore cannot store any of the above mentioned essentials. Ironically, the brain cannot function without these essential elements either.

- In normal arteries, oxygen rich blood flows smoothly. The arteries remain flexible, and therefore are considered normal.

- Cholesterol and plaque accumulates over time in our arteries, and get stuck or lodged to the inner walls of our arteries.

- The arteries become narrow and this causes the blood flow to get restricted. This causes blood to spurt (somewhat similar to capillary action in the air-conditioning system where the condensed gas passes through a very thin tube (capillary) thereby increasing its pressure therein)

- Blood flow with some pressure behind it continuously hits the walls of the clogged arteries, which causes rupture. Clogged arteries are when plaque is formed on the inside of the arteries. Spurting of blood with high pressure behind it dislodges some of the plaque. These blood particles clump together and a blood clot is formed

- A blood clot can further reduce the flow of blood through an artery, or can completely block passage of blood through it. A blood clot in the heart causes a Heart Attack, and a blood clot in the Brain is called a Stroke or a Brain Attack. Briefly, in a heart attack the blood supply to the heart is reduced or blocked, and in a stroke blood supply to the brain is reduced or stopped. Although heart attacks and strokes can cause death without warning, heart patients in most cases suffer less or no negative effects to their brain and other parts of the body. However, stroke patients suffer significant damage to the brain as well as other affected parts of the body. The root causes are similar but the effects are somewhat different.

It is natural for our bodies to create blood clots to stop excessive bleeding from a cut on our bodies. When we cut ourselves we bleed, and consequently various particles in our blood form a blood clot to stop bleeding, which is a natural process, Formation of blood clots can also occur if the plaque in the arteries is broken or ruptured. In both cases, blood clots form causing to reduce the flow of blood, or completely blocking it to various parts of the body.

According to Center for Disease Control (CDC)

- more than 900,000 people die of Cardio Vascular Disease in the USA, each year,

- Stroke is the third leading cause of death in America

- more than 100 deaths occur from stroke and heart disease every hour

- One in five adults has some form of Cardio Vascular Disease (CVD)

- Stroke is the leading cause of Disability

- many survivors never recover

- 20% of Stroke victims require Institutional Care

An estimated $394 Billions were spent on CVD related health care in 2005, and about $242 Billions were spent in healthcare cost, and $152 Billions in lost productivity. Medicare spends about $26 Billion in CVD related Hospitalization cost each year.

90% of Middle Aged Americans will develop High Blood Pressure in their life time, and 70% who have it now do not have it controlled. Without adequate measures to prevent Strokes or Heart Attacks will result in a sharp rise in American death rate from it, and a steep rise in "survivors with dependency of one kind or another".

It was around middle of spring in 1996 when I experienced unusually difficult set of let downs and breach of trust related circumstances, one after another. So my anxiety, worries, anger, and feeling of being a victim were very high, otherwise, I was in an excellent health with no history of Headaches, ever.

Being under stress and anger, one late night I developed a crucifying headache. I ignored it and went to bed to shut myself off. I woke up early in the morning, the pain was still there. I put both of my hands on each side of my head, and held them for a couple of minutes, thinking the pain will ease. My hands got moist. I thought it was sweat. To my surprise, it was not sweat; it was blood on my left hand which lead me to think that I must have scratched myself during the course of night. I was dizzy from the headache, but never felt less than a Macho who could handle anything and everything. I proceeded to do my morning chores by brushing my teeth, shaving, etc. I noticed that some blood was oozing from a swollen opening which was on my left temple. The opening was about one eighth of an inch in diameter, raised, with somewhat shattered skin around the opening. Blood had dried there and it was still drying. While rinsing my mouth, I spitted blood, a lot of it. I drank a lot of water, but dizziness continued, and I felt that I was losing energy levels, so I took a few minutes' rest after each activity. I blamed this weakness to mal-nutrition. So, I ate a big steak with couple of eggs to boost my strength and energy, took vitamin supplements, and went to my vegetable garden and worked the soil for a few hours just to get rid off this weakness and awesome feeling of which I had no prior experience, ever. I felt weak and experienced no energy whatsoever. In fact, I had a compelling desire to lie down somewhere quick.

No one should ever attempt to do this which is awfully wrong. I did not know the exact meaning of stroke. I had always associated it with the heat stroke of which I had heard about but never experienced, or knew much about it. Ignorance has never been proven to be a good excuse. I paid for my ignorance by creating a condition to have a stroke, and then not knowing about it, and then by playing tough with myself. I should have taken aspirin and rested for several days very quietly, that is, in the absence of medical help.

I stayed active against all odds, and was determined to get out of this phase of weakness. Either that evening, or the next evening, my next door neighbor, a nurse, saw me walking and she asked what had happened to my legs. My legs were wobbling. She commented on my face which was flushed and did not look normal. I thought I was explaining like I always had but she could not understand most of it.... She told me that I had had a STROKE, and I should call my doctor immediately. I was in a complete disbelief. I carried a strong feeling in my mind that "these things don't happen to me and can't happen to me." I did not have any assigned and designated doctor because I thought that I would visit one when I needed one. I maintained health insurance, though, but did not know that without having a designated doctor I would be denied emergency medical help. I was told that was the rule at that time. Any how I called the telephone number for emergency on the back of my Health Insurance. Card This took me to another unchartered experience.

For health emergency 800 numbers did not ring in the facility I used to visit for my annual checkups, but it rang about 60-70 miles away somewhere in Maryland or Virginia, and several hours were spent being interviewed by a few nurses who kept me on the phone for several hours. I could not be admitted for Emergency Treatment, because I did not have a Designated Physician, even though I paid my premiums regularly on time. I was advised that it was the law at that time, and whether I was in good health or not I should have had a designated personal physician on their file. After a lot of aggravating conversation, nurses agreed to bring me in This Healthcare provider's nursing staff who was receiving Emergency Health calls DID NOT KNOW the general area of Greater Baltimore & Washington, along the I-95 corridor. As a result of this, they offered me Emergency Facility in Silver Spring, about 60 miles from my home that is if I could drive down there. It was about 8.30 pm, and of course I never had the brains to call an Ambulance, because I did not know how the Healthcare System worked. Again, this was due to my ignorance.

After realizing a bit more about the geographical details, these good nurses advised me that they had booked me in a hospital in Havre de Grace, about 20 miles from my home then. Even though, I was weak, insecure, and desperate, I just wanted to be sure that I would be accepted. So I called this hospital, and they acknowledged that my Healthcare provider had called, and I should bring a check for $20, 000.. I was agitated. They felt the need to accommodate me, so they dropped the amount to $15,000.I hung up by yelling "I will get better myself" That was the end of my treatment at that point. After that I experienced at least two more strokes, and each one of them produced blood from the outside of the head as well as from the inside. I experienced several minor strokes after that. Each time, I experienced various kinds of weaknesses, disabilities, disorientation, vision problems, reading problems, walking problems, speech difficulties, coordination problems, pain in joints, etc., etc. I felt compelled to take rest, and I learnt to take rest and eat nutritious non fat foods with lots of water every day. I did not like to continue taking aspirin every day, because I thought that it might give me ulcers later, which was an unconfirmed fact in my mind.

My neighbor had advised me to drink some wine instead if I did not feel comfortable with taking aspirin. So, every evening before dinner only I drank two glasses of red wine. In the beginning I tried it with water to get accustomed to its taste and acidity. It worked. I feel lucky that each time I had a stroke, significant or a small one, the blood did come out of the damaged blood vessel; possibly it drained in to my stomach, some came out of my mouth, nose. During the first three strokes, blood came out from outside of my head as well as from the inside of my head. Subsequent strokes occur when adequate attention and care are not given to the patient, or like in my case, the patient was so careless that similar stroke causing acts were repeated over and over again. I was repeating the same business endeavors with different business partners, and getting hurt successively in the same manner while continuously maintaining a disposition of strong, worldly, knowledgeable, and professional business executive. I also learned that after any physical activity like walking a relatively long distance, I experienced a mild headache which stayed with me for a day or so, thereafter I used to see some pink color in my mucus for several days with sustained weakness and lifelessness. After a few days this pink color used to disappear. But, for sure, each time I exerted myself beyond a certain limit I suffered some headache and then mild bleeding for several days. Sometime, small pieces of dried blood came out of my nose, and less dried blood from my throat. Symptoms and outcomes remained consistent, and I learned new things on a regular basis. Some of the things were never to get involved in discussions, arguments, or question and answer sessions with any one. Also, I learned that to get better I had to relearn everything again, and in order to accomplish that I would have to face myself making a lot of mistakes on hourly basis. I was making a lot of foul ups in the neighborhood and in the marketplace due to various disabilities I had developed, and this behavior was rewarding me with unbearable humiliation on daily basis.

To get better in a new place where people did not know me at all started to occupy my mind on a regular basis. I tried out my capabilities by driving long distance gradually making stops every 10 miles at first. Of course, the idea was to make errors far away from home, where no one knew me. This worked, and I graduated. After several difficult attempts of decision making and public relations challenges, I found a new residence about 60 miles away. Moving to a new residence was somewhat hectic and laborious, and that evening I experienced sustained headache and then some bleeding, which made me lie down most of every day for about 10 days period. By this time, I had learned what was happening and what needed to be done. Each time headache is felt, I know instantly that I need to sit down and take rest until the headache is gone. Any delays in taking rest immediately after sensing the oncoming headache, causes lifelessness and sustained weakness for many days, and until the dried out blood comes out through my nose or mouth I remain in the same condition. These are small strokes which I have experienced several times over a period of 10 years. Now, I know how to recognize the oncoming small stroke and how to handle it, besides maintaining dietary and lifestyle changes. Now for more than a year I have not experienced even a small stroke, though occasionally I felt I was near getting a severe headache.

Interestingly, before the sensation of oncoming headache there are signals of slow down in the body functions, energy levels, uneasiness, and physical instability. The best action would be to recognize these feelings or symptoms and then take precautions like taking an aspirin, resting, and taking it easy for several hours. Although it is hard to sense such feelings or symptoms when one is deeply engrossed in day to day work, yet learning about it and focusing on it could prove to be priceless. Now, I am able to recognize the signals of getting a headache and am able to avoid the experience of having another one. Under stressful or tiresome conditions, which should be avoided by all of us, I have felt the sensation of an oncoming headache which signals me to stop whatever I am doing, go home, take an aspirin, change thoughts, and lie down for a while. It works each time, and I strongly recommend you to do this, even if you have never had any stroke or heart condition before, because it may prevent you from having one.

I was causing my own strokes by not resting after the first one, and giving up the struggle until my health allowed me to do so. Competitiveness, ego, pugnacity, anger, and restitution should be given up immediately after the first stroke; otherwise probability for having another stroke becomes very high if not a certain one In fact, if we adopt this attitude in the first place, we can prevent having a stroke altogether. I learned the hard way something very important which I would like to share with the readers, and hope they consider using this method just as soon as they get the feeling of the on coming stroke. In previous pages, I made an attempt to describe the symptoms of stroke that are recognizable. When those symptoms appear, it is already too late. Each one of us should acquaint ourselves with the symptoms of the pre-sensation of the oncoming of a stroke, or a heart attack. Your personal physician should be consulted for such symptoms.

From my experience of stroke, I learned that about 2 to 3 days before, a feeling of tiredness for no reason, difficulty in concentration or focusing on any one subject, sustained feeling of lying down somewhere, sitting on a chair does not provide the satisfying feeling of rest, acuteness of vision is reduced, prefer to be alone than being with other people, noise seem to be more bothersome than before, difficulty in shaking off the thoughts in the mind, a feeling that a lot of thoughts have been accumulated in the mind and have not been processed, mind seems to be over crowded, a sensation of headache yet no headache, using hands and arms seem to be weaker than before, effort to clench fists does not seem to be inviting, etc. These mild symptoms of the on coming stroke should be recognized by everyone above 50 years of age, and others as well because stroke does strike people in their twenties. This is a kind of warning that the system may be shut down. At this time, the best thing you can do is to stop all activities, including being near people, and follow these steps. Take an aspirin or a substitute with at least one glass of water at room temperature or a bit warmer. First sit down on a chair and close your eyes, ears, and mouth. This means that you are not taking in any additional information inside your brain for now. Brain never stops to function. Let the brain keep the information which is already there, and process it. In fact, you have just started to slow down the brain activity, which is very important at this stage. After sometime being in the chair, lie down with your face up. Under such circumstances, I lie down on my back flat on the carpet. Stay in that position for some time, and try to move your thoughts to some pleasant arena of good life, good friends, travel, etc. If you do this just for a day or two, you will come out without the occurrence of stroke entirely. Even if the odds happen to be against you due to some other health conditions or home environmental circumstances, and you end up experiencing a stroke, the stroke will be of minor variety. Taking an aspirin and calling your doctor should always be considered.

Minor variety stroke in my vocabulary is when I feel dizzy, lifeless, energy less, limp, and with difficulties in focus and vision, etc. and want to lie down somewhere all the time. This basically means that somewhere in the brain blood was not flowing properly due to a blood clot which partially blocked the blood flow. If such is the case, then the blood clot will clear out in a few days, either with the help of a physician or by doing the right things on your own. If you are careful with your diet and drink a lot of water, take an aspirin, rest a lot, and maintain stable state of mind, the clot will either get dissolved or exit through your sinuses, or the bile will carry it out of the body. This lasts about 10 days or more, but it is a good warning sign to be careful. Once the clot is out, the feeling of good health arrives almost instantly, even though the weakness lingers on for a few days. Until the brain is free of the clot the stroke condition will remain and deteriorate on a daily basis, no matter how insignificant the stroke might be. After the first few major strokes I suffered many minor strokes which were the result of carelessness, not taking sufficient rest, not eating nutritious meals at the right time, not controlling anger, and repeating the same things which brought the stroke condition in the first place. After a major stroke, any exertion or fatigue can bring on a stroke. A potential stroke or a heart patient, with or without prior history, has got to be careful and responsible every day to stay healthy. Now, during this stroke sensation period, after taking aspirin or substitute, and resting for a while, you do not feel comfortable, do visit your doctor. I think you will be fine if you stay engaged, and stay on top of this issue of your well being.

HEART DISEASE

To recognize the precursors of Heart Attack, the sensation is a bit different, even though most of the underlying causes are the same as that of stroke condition. As a young boy and later as a young adult, I witnessed various phases of heart condition within my own immediate family. Majority of males members from my mother's and father's side suffered from heart attacks, and quite many died in their fifty's. I watched them go through all the phases of heart disease, including death by it. So, I learned to recognize various symptoms, if not all, of people with heart condition, and how close they could be from a heart attack. Genes do play a major role in our life, especially in health related conditions. A few times, I did experience being just seconds away from having a heart attack and death. My past experience of being a member of family of heart patients had made me somewhat alert to certain precursors to heart attack. At certain times, I felt that I was a minute or two away from having a heart attack, and other times my feeling was that it was going to happen any second. Quite a terrifying state to be in, especially when you are living alone and the time is between 2.00 am and 6.00 am. At that time, getting out of the bed when I was in deep sleep is a clear demonstration that there is an innate protective system within our bodies and the brain, which gives out alerts to save ourselves from a calamity, whether it is internal or external.

There are numerous kinds of HEART disease, and new names will emerge through the on going research in this field. There are a few major kinds of heart attacks which are described below to provide an over all view of this severe health problem.

STABLE ANGINA occurs when excessive exertion or demanding activity is carried out. Athletics, snow shoveling in the spring time, swimming, etc. This is also known as or predictable Angina.

UNSTABLE ANGINA occurs when there is severe pain in the chest, which is caused when there is not enough supply of blood to the heart.

Reduced supply of blood to the heart is caused by narrowing of the arteries. It is painful, causes the patient to sweat, and feel dizzy.

CONGENITAL HEART BLOCKAGE occurs when there is some interference in the electrical nerve impulses which regulate the rhythmic pumping activity of the heart muscle. When the two upper chambers of the heart beat normally, but the two lower chambers of the heart lag behind and are out of sync, or beat abnormally. Several other conditions are related to it including abnormal formation of heart or major blood vessels.

CORONARY HEART DISEASE is best described when the coronary arteries become narrow due to the formation of plaque within the arterial walls, and cause stoppage or reduce the flow of blood to the heart muscle, which, in most cases, results in a heart attack.

HEART FAILURE occurs when the heart muscles fail to pump as much blood as the body needs. Our body responds to this emergency of short supply of blood by taking protective measures. Our body increases the heart rate, the size of the heart is increased, also conserves the salt and water to increase the quantity of blood in the blood stream. These are emergency measures taken by the body, but it lasts only for a very short time.

Just after the heart attack, most surviving patients will feel lifeless which is similar to stroke patients, however, heart patients have almost no adverse effects in the functioning of the brain and most of the limbs. Irritability, combativeness, anger, restlessness, short tempered, disagreements, dissatisfaction, etc are some very prominent personality traits I witnessed in my family members after they suffered a heart attack.

HEART ATTACK occurs due to the plaque formation inside of the coronary artery wall, which results in weakened and damaged cells below the plaque. This damage can cause to develop a leakage which allows the LDL to enter inside the arterial wall. Once inside the arterial wall, LDL gets oxidized which is toxic and body's protective mechanism comes in to play. A lump of various elements in the blood stream rush to the leaking spot to block it, and a lump is formed, which is known as plaque. Plaque can break loose or break open and travel to other parts of the coronary artery. This break away piece of plaque can damage many locations within the coronary artery, and more plaque is formed. Artery becomes narrower. Also, broken plaque provides signal to platelets to move in and a blood clot is formed. This newly formed blood clot can become bigger by accumulating other substances in the blood stream as it travels and can block the blood flow to the heart, resulting in heart attack.

Most of the heart attacks are experienced by people between the ages of 35 and 65. Lowering overall cholesterol levels, especially LDL, can prevent heart attack or stroke. It is estimated that about 3% of all LDL in the body is oxidized for one reason or another, and it poses continuous risk. By lowering the total LDL, the probability factor for the LDL to enter the arterial walls will be greatly reduced. If this probability is maintained then the already formed plaque inside the arterial walls would not get aggravated by the oxidized LDL. Another precaution is by intake of vitamin E which can improve the health of arterial wall lining. Therefore, lowering the LDL levels in the blood stream and the regular intake of vitamin E can greatly reduce the risk factor of experiencing a heart attack or a stroke.

Over the years, I experienced several incidents when I got up from the bed and gasping for air, with my eyes closed in the night. At times, I came out in my pajamas to the balcony of my apartment in icy cold sub zero temperatures, and stayed there for some time inhaling and exhaling through my mouth. I could not breathe from my nostrils during those moments. At the same time, my hand used to reach and rub frantically just below the left rib cage where the heart is supposed to be located. I used to feel an acute feeling of tightness, like a painful muscle knot or a cramp, just below the rib cage toward the center. It was an awful feeling and experience which gave me a sensation that I was going away. Some strange feeling compelled me to keep on rubbing at that spot for an hour to three hours.

The only time I stopped rubbing was to open the aspirin bottle cap, which required both hands because the bottle had a children proof cap. The secondary aspect of this experience was that within 15 to 30 minutes, while I was still rubbing, I had a sensation of weakness and tingling traveling from my left shoulder to the arm up to the wrist. Fear entered my mind at this stage, and I rubbed below the left rib cage more and more until I could breathe from my nostrils again. After several hours I felt stable, but breathless, scared, tired, and fearful to return to bed. My face remained flushed with some kind of a glow for a few days. I analyzed and reanalyzed each experience several times, and came to realize and learn a few lessons for myself. I would like to share some highlights of these lessons with the readers, with the hope that some day they might prove to be helpful to someone living alone and who did not know what to do under similar circumstances.

I practice to this day what these near heart attack incidents taught me, of course with the exception of certain days. I learned that I should eat dinner before 7.00 pm on a regular basis, which is about 3 hours prior to going to bed. If for some reasons the dinner is late, then make the bedtime to be late as well. I love to eat a lot, but I have reduced the portions of my meals. Instead, I eat something little all day. If and when there is some kind of meat in my dinner menu, then I make sure that it is just a token or in a very small portion. Meat takes longer to travel downward. I walk after dinner each day, and then get involved in activities before going to bed on time. Before going to bed each night I make sure that I am as calm and peaceful as I can manage to be. I have stopped going to bed in an agitated state of mind. If I feel agitated during the middle of the night, I get up and sit on the chair, watch TV or do nothing, until I feel stabilized enough to go to bed again. An important lesson I learned and that is never to sleep late in the morning. I always get up early in the morning even after a few hours of sleep. I can always take a nap or two during the day time. But getting up early is a good thing because most of the heart attacks and strokes occur during that time. Once you are up and out of bed, only after a pause of a minute or more, the probability of an occurrence of stroke or heart attack becomes much lower. Now, I have developed a kind of habit to get out of bed, no matter what time it may be, if I have slightest sensation of the oncoming discomfort in breathing, in the head, or just a leg cramp. I have learned that this is the best way to tackle a situation like this, because I believe that one does not have to be sleeping when something goes wrong with the heart or the brain. If you are up you can do something about the problem. There is no chance whatsoever to be able to do anything to save yourself if you happen to be in bed or sleeping.

I like the ideas of Dr. Bob Arnold who suggests in his book (Seven steps to stop heart attack) that all patients should be prepared for heart attack. Calling 911 procedures, selection of the right hospital, ambulance response time, details of medications, LDL/HDL levels, current details on allergies and medication intake, and results of tests and screenings should be kept handy.

This suggestion appeals to me the most primarily because my father died of heart attack due to the delay in accessing medical help in time. I remember rushing out in my pajamas and slippers at 10.00 PM during winter time to the doctor's house just one block away, and shaking his gate while yelling for help. Hearing my voice people from adjoining houses came to help me to draw doctor's attention. The doctor was reluctant to come out in cold and it took him 50 minutes to reach our house, and exactly on his arrival my father died at age 51. Another example on similar lines was when my uncle suffered from a heart attack at age 50, an ambulance arrived on time, picked him up and could not take him to the hospital in time because the ambulance had run out gas. My uncle died in the ambulance which had to travel a long distance to reach my uncle's house, with no gas left to return. Therefore, it is prudent to have all the emergency details ready for the possibility of such an occurrence. If feasible, patients should make a choice to live within the vicinity of a hospital to minimize delays in receiving emergency medical help.

Also, I suggest that each morning upon waking when you are ready to get up from your bed, take a few moments to get up to reach the sitting position on the edge of the bed. Again, take several moments before getting on your feet from the sitting position. Even better would be to sit on the edge of the bed and contemplate the agenda you are going to have for the day. Or you may like to pray a little bit. You must have some prayer in your mind. If you do not know any prayer then make one up which speaks of your heart's desires. The simplest prayer any one can have is to be 'thankful to god, or the universe, or the nature." You can also choose to thank your parents who provided you with the opportunity to experience life, and who ceaselessly cared for you, fed you, clothed you, sent you to school, comforted you, and took care of you in every possible manner, never stopped loving you until the last breath they took before departing from this world.

Another idea to pray is to ask for good health without which everything is morbid and gray. You may choose to reflect on your life path, various experiences, children and relatives, friends, or some subject of interest, coming birthdays, anniversaries, festivals, etc. This kind of brief contemplation will most likely set your day, and the mood. Your mood will pave a path for the types of activities you would like to participate in. It will also provide with the positive thoughts and look forwardness to get on the agenda. Each morning before getting out of your bed, sitting on the edge of the bed for a few minutes contemplating, praying, or meditating, or just thinking of things to do during the day should become a routine not just for the stroke or heart attack patients but for everybody. It will prove to be extremely healthful in several ways.

This daily routine may prove to be very beneficial to you in the long run, and may even save your life. Getting up from the bed in a kind of frenzy could put the heart and the brain in a very stressful state, and that is a big transition from an extreme resting position to an active one. During resting and sleeping positions, the heart rate and the body temperature drops, and pulling yourself out of this position should be a slow process. Just observe athletes who warm up before participating in any exercise. Even before the warm ups, they require months of practicing, sometime every day, to reach that level. There are athletes who do otherwise, do go to the hospital in an ambulance either from the sports field or soon after. This very same thing should be observed when doing something strenuous while in a sitting position or standing position with movement. During a movement, the normal functions of the body are active, and this poses a less dangerous situation for most of the people. The best is to avoid doing strenuous tasks if you are not active and in shape, and if you do end up in a situation where you have got to do something like this, then move your body limbs for a few minutes and thereafter carry out the task as slowly as you can. Therefore, do make the process of getting up from your bed a slow one, because otherwise you will be putting your body to an extreme stress within a matter of few seconds.

Another very important suggestion I would like to pass on to you is to check with your doctor if you are flight worthy before taking a plane ride. Fluctuation of cabin pressure and sudden changes in the aircraft altitude levels can make the blood in the body rush from one side to other in a matter of seconds, and if there are some remaining weak or unhealed spots in the brain, heart, or in the arteries, the consequences can be devastating. Here, again prevention will prove to be better than cure.

You are probably aware of the fact that heart attack is similar to stroke or brain attack. Heart attack occurs when coronary arteries are blocked. Coronary arteries supply oxygen rich blood to the heart. The blockage is caused by Plaque built up, and when the plaque breaks loose or opens up blood clots form around it, which results in partial blockage or total blockage of the coronary artery or arteries. Heart muscles die if oxygen and nutrients rich blood supply is reduced or stopped. If a large area of heart is affected by the cut off of blood supply, then instant death occurs. Therefore heart attack patients require immediate help. Symptoms of heart attack are pain in or around the heart, pain is traveling to the shoulders and arms, neck, jaws, and the back, sweating, vomiting, difficulty in breathing, general weakness, and numbness, etc.

There are numerous indirect indicators of heart disease. Pain in the chest, pain in the back just below the left shoulder blade and toward the middle, muscle cramps in the calf, thigh, arm, chest, abdomen are some of the indicators, however, there is another very important indicator which is often ignored. If you have thickened nails which are difficult to clip, and if some of the nails have bluish spots at the root, or if the nails seem to be curved over the end, especially the finger nails, then it should be taken as the problem with blood circulation, atherosclerosis, and heart disease. If the finger nails are curving around the ends then it could be indicator of advanced stages of heart disease. The moment you notice these indicators, start taking dietary and other healthful lifestyle measures right away. If your blood test show abnormalities then probably your doctor will advise you the treatment you would need, however, if this happens not to be the case then you should take all the necessary steps on your own. Your own steps could be right diet, exercise, state of mind, freedom from stress, etc., etc. You do not want to celebrate good health because the doctor cleared you and gave a clean bill of health. Suppose he is wrong. My neighbor, a senior lady went to have regular check up and received a clean bill of health from her doctor. Within the same hour, she dropped dead of unknown causes. Of course, old age was the alibi, and doctors never guarantee immortality.Watch and manage your own symptoms, and take full advantage of your doctor's advice.

CHAPTER III

CAUSES & CURES OF STROKE & HEART DISEASE

- Control high blood pressure and manage it by your self

- Control high blood cholesterol and manage it by your self

- Learn to recognize signs and symptoms and decide when to call 911

- Improve emergency resources

- Improve quality of care, choice of caregiver, medical facility, and monitor it

- Control risk factors, and make sure to monitor and manage it by yourself.

- Self manage prevention of Strokes and Heart Disease, and you can do it.

- Take charge of your well being

- Manage your health and any ailments that you are suffering from.

CONTROLLING YOUR BLOOD PRESSURE

- 65 million Americans have High Blood Pressure

- Additionally 59 million are Hypertensive

- 70% of people with High Blood Pressure do not have it under control

- Just lowering your blood pressure by 12 points, you can greatly reduce the probability of having stroke or heart attack. Breathing exercises, changing the state of mind, reducing irritability and anger, eating healthy diet in small portions, adoption of regular walking and light exercise routine, having proper sleep, etc. can bring your blood pressure down. With lower blood pressure, you will feel much better besides reducing the chances of stroke or heart attack.

DIET: eat vegetables, fruits, legumes, nuts, low to non fat diet, and other foods containing phytochemicals within the guidelines of your doctor. Some information is provided to inform the stroke and heart patients about the foods, vitamins, nutritional values, etc. later in this book. This information will help the patient to understand why a certain food should be consumed regularly, and why certain foods should be consumed occasionally if not avoided completely. Also, such a brief introduction will help the patient to learn to read the food labels and assess the beneficial as well as the risk factors of specific foods.

EXERCISE: walk daily as much as you can, and participate in some light exercise routine which you can easily maintain on a regular basis. The exercise must be very light to start with. Strenuous exercise and too much manipulation of body muscles in a short time just after the stroke or heart attack could prove to be stressful and could tear the muscles, tendons, or ligaments. At this time, the body is extremely fragile, just like a baby, and everything inside is weak and delicate. I personally experienced this weakness just after the first and subsequent strokes, and learned the hard way. Because I was maintaining a mind set that nothing serious happened to me and I was as strong as before, I tried to carry out exercises which should never have been attempted by anyone in that condition. I ate cholesterol and fat laden foods to get stronger quickly, tried to dig up my garden to gain strength and energy in a short time, and carried out stomach crunches while my face and other parts of my body were still numb from the effects of stroke. All this without the help of a doctor, or anyone's advice, resulted in swollen wrists, severe pain in the elbows, knees, ankles, neck, and later broken stomach lining resulting in Inguinal hernia.

These were very painful experiences which lasted for a long time. Inguinal hernia is when stomach lining breaks allowing a portion of intestine to come out of the protective support layer thereby creating a small bulge. This condition, if not rectified, can cause a host of life threatening problems. Therefore, all walking body movements, and exercise should be carried out with extreme caution. Even if the doctor or caregiver suggests you to carry out something physical, you must use your own judgment for each of such actions. It is your body, and you know its strengths and weaknesses better than anyone else. Learn to say no as often as you can manage to do so. Later in the book you will read my own experience about my stress test under my doctor's advice, which could have sent me to surgical table needlessly. A few months ago a neighbor and friend ended up breathing heavily after some physical exertion. To make sure he was not in any danger he checked with his healthcare provider who gave him stress test and found clogged arteries in his body. At age 82 he went through triple bypass surgery.

Do stress tests create compelling procedural circumstances which demand triple bypass surgery? Is it safe for the patient to be in the middle of two very strong and powerful entities; one is the medical community and the other is insurance companies? Medical community has the life saving tools and capability, while the insurance companies have the money. Medical community wants that money from the insurance companies, and they can get only through you as patient who is in the middle. Now if you get sick and get treated or counseled, the medical community gets paid. If you get well and stop receiving medical help then medical community does not get paid. They will continue to get paid as long as you remain sick and seek their help. The medical community gets paid only after they treat the patients. In normal life, you do not get paid for the work which was not done, done wrongly, or which created another damage, etc. and the work performer will either correct it or replace it to receive the payment. In the provision of healthcare, this is not the case. The medical community gets paid no matter what the outcome may be, at least in most of the cases. And who knows about the level of expertise a particular doctor has. I remember that I could not draft a decent letter after graduating from college. Could a similar situation exist in the medical community? During my normal checkups over the years, I have encountered medical professionals who did not know much about the job they were assigned to do. Who has enough time to fight a lawsuit and who can guarantee if the patient is going to benefit from such an endeavor? Seniors who have just a few active years of life left wouldn't want to spend their precious years in fighting anyone, nor should they choose to make medical visits and consuming prescription drugs as a way of life because that is not living a life.

About 90% of all American adults have some level of clogged arteries in their body. Just see how much potential of bypass surgeries and rehab is there-worth billions of dollars. There are many other high potential areas in surgery, medications, and cures. All these potentials will materialize if people keep getting sick and keep the dependency of staying healthy on someone else. So the alternative is to avoid unnecessary medical visits and treatment, medical errors, and unsatisfactory medical response to your specific ailment by staying healthy on your own and limiting use of medical help to the minimum. Remember that healthcare profession is a business, and as long as they keep receiving new patients and old patients on a regular basis they will prosper in their business. It is in your own interest to stay healthy on your own, and provide medical community the opportunity to make money as rarely as possible. Besides staying healthy, it will save you money as a patient and as a taxpayer.

After the stroke or heart attack, we must pay special attention to the needs of FEMALE and MALE patients specifically. Females are gentler, delicate, and require more privacy than male patients. Even though medical treatment may be the same for both sexes, but due to inherent social structures which have been established thousands of years ago require females to be treated a bit differently. Here comes the judgment call on the part of health provider, and discretion must be applied to the process of such medical treatment, which includes a variety of specialized attention to females. The perception of males toward females is much different than that of females toward men. Females are mothers, who raised both boys and girls, and therefore they can tolerate males being exposed in an otherwise private disposition, and to which males generally would not emphatically object to. However, females may feel awkward and stressful being witnessed or watched in a similarly private but awkward disposition, and consequently may shy away from the treatment or become averse to any procedure in those circumstances. Therefore social conditions that the patients have been accustomed to, within the social structure as established by the culture, become very important for the cure and fast healing of the patient. No patient should feel that they are being tossed and shuffled around disregarding their gender, social status, even educational and financial background. I would not accept sharing a hospital room with another undesirable (according to my own evaluation) patient. I would resent it every minute. Of course, under unconscious state, no patient knows the location he or she has been hauled to, but when the consciousness returns the scene should be acceptable for the well being of the patient.

Very important thing I got to know is to AVOID isometric exercises at all costs. Isometric exercise means creating a muscle tension without the motion of the body. Kinetic exercise means creating muscle tension with the motion of the body. Isometric exercises can raise the blood pressure to dangerously high levels thereby creating equally high pressure on the cardiac system within a very short time. Movement of the body during exercise pumps blood regularly to the muscles being used. However, when there is no movement of the body, blood is not being pumped to meet the sudden increase in demand of the muscles in tension. It is dangerous for people who start exercise without warm up, or who do not usually use those muscles on a regular basis, or who are weak and not in shape, etc. Exercises requiring sudden effort, or sudden in put of strength should be avoided completely. It is believed that President Eisenhower suffered a heart attack when he tried to dislodge a stuck window. A lot of people suffer from heart attacks; even die, from trying to do sudden muscle strain causing activities and exercises. Many years ago, a close friend of mine volunteered to push someone's stalled car so that it could get started. He was 28 years old body builder in very good health. From a standing position he started to push the car when felt a sudden chest pain, and suffered a massive heart attack. He did not live to reach the hospital in time. While living in the Snow Belt, after the first heavy snow fall, it is common for the people to remove snow from their driveways and sidewalks late that night or the next morning. You could hear the sound of shovels scratching the pavements in every neighborhood. Also, you could hear the occasional siren of approaching ambulance in some neighborhoods. In the same vein, just as soon as the spring breaks in the snow belt regions, joggers start jogging after several months of inactivity, and a lot of them are taken to the hospitals for Cardio Vascular related health problems. Bringing sudden strain to the body muscles and creating an excessive flow of blood in a specific area within a very short time can cause severe health problems. So try your level best to avoid such experiences.

In most cases and under healthful circumstances, regular and moderate exercise produces much better results for the individual to prevent stroke or heart disease than otherwise. At the same time, we must consider a fact that human body is not a perfect body in the clinical sense. We come in to this world with strengths and weaknesses in our body, and this applies to almost all the individuals. While exceptions are there, may be 1% or more in the human population which could be identified as being completely normal with no physical weaknesses, but there are definitely identifiable weaknesses in the general population. The degree and type of these weaknesses vary with each individual. When we exert ourselves in the arena of sports, work place, or just walking fast in a sustained manner over a period of time, the physical weakness will emerge, for which medical help will be needed without a doubt. Most of us are aware of the fact that athletes develop a variety of problems with legs, ankles, muscles, etc. and similarly the scientists, lab researchers, librarians, proof readers, pilots, etc. end up developing problems with their vision. I know this because I have been involved in sports and athletics, later in jogging and now in walking only, which brings me to confirm that heavy and demanding use of bones, muscles and organs do take toll on the body and consequently various health problems emerge, specifically in over exerted areas of the body, at one time or another in life. What I am trying to say is that there is an optimal level of use of each organ, muscle, ligament, tendon, joint, etc. in our body, and if we continuously pound on them or over exert them, they are bound to develop some problems which will require medical help. Once these problems related to over exerting our body emerge, they never seem to go away also. It leads us to say that by over exertion, the existing physical weaknesses get elevated to a much higher level, which we can do without. The physical weakness which was not bothering us before and we could live with it, has been developed to a noticeable and problematic degree. Excessive and strenuous exercises are not good for majority of people. On the other hand, low impact, less or moderately strenuous and sustainable exercises are much better. Better exercises are those which can be carried out throughout your life. In view of this thought, stoke or heart attack patient is required to be extra careful in the exercise agenda.

STATE OF MIND: Be peaceful, loving, and friendly, even though your faculties for these functions are damaged. It may be easier said than done, because after the stroke, all emotions and responses get disorganized due to a variety of damages inside the brain. It does not become easy to be peaceful, loving, or friendly. In fact, the condition is quite opposite to these traits. On a drop of a nickel one can become irritated and obnoxious, primarily because of memory loss which partially disabled the patient.

Patients do tend to look friendly which is because the patient needs help and sympathy which become in short supply, because people cannot understand what the patient is saying or wants. Moreover, in today's world people do not want to be friendly with stroke or heart patients who are unable to participate in life, socially as well as economically, and fear that they might get stuck for no satisfying reason. Modern age is different, and patient must accept such a social environment when everyone wants to maximize benefits from each hour of the day especially for their own satisfaction. Stroke and heart patients do not necessarily provide any incentives of good company, or stimulating social life. Patients seem to lose the capability to maintain the membership of the club known as society, and eventually get dropped out. Also, in the process of seeking help and sympathy, patient exposes herself or himself to a grave danger of fraud. Uncouth people can make the patient sign on financial and legal papers, etc. resulting in loss of savings and assets, primarily due to the fact that reasoning and analytical capabilities are diminished or at their minimum level.

Often, patients expect to hear from loved ones, friends, and acquaintances and in many cases the call becomes a source of confidence, encouragement, and being loved. However, each phone call takes a toll on the patient. Phone calls can make the patient irritable and annoyed because the patient cannot retain what was heard, unable to process the words and the information, and is unable to form words in time to respond appropriately. In short the patient is not completely fit to communicate and this causes a difficulty in patient's mind, which leads him or her to be annoyed and irritated. I found that my business friends would only call me when they were in the car. Voice on the mobile phone was never clear all the time and the wide variation in the voice levels used to make it very difficult for me to completely understand the conversation. Therefore my participation was just saying 'yes, alright,' which gave me a great deal of discomfort. Wanting to receive their favors and to be on the good side, I had to listen to them. The mobile phone calls used to last for a long time and I found myself on my land phone for a long time each day which was extremely tiresome. For some reason all these business friends would not take my calls in their offices. After quite a long time I learned that all these business friends were passing their driving time on the phone with me, harvesting valuable information about my client base, advising my clients that they were taking care of me, and rendering me useless at the same time. Some people need to stay occupied while driving, and they find people who are always available because of some health condition that warrants them to stay home.

Patients become easy targets of so many people with dubious intentions. I learned an important lesson which is very important for stroke and heart disease patients that is to avoid answering phone calls which you think is from the cell phone, unless you know for sure that the person who is calling from a cell phone is genuinely caring. Secondly, let most of the calls go to your voice mail box and this will provide you with the convenience to call the right person when it is convenient for you to call. Also, this delay will give you sufficient time to prepare your conversation. Make this a routine until you are healed, because it will reduce the irritability and annoyance which causes serious delays in the healing process. Also it will provide you with some protection from people who want to take undue advantage of you while you are in this difficult and non functional state of physical and mental health.

ACCEPTANCE: occurrence of stroke or heart attack cannot and should not be denied; it should be accepted and verbalized. Unless such grave experience is accepted, it will be difficult to heal the effects of it and to get better in a timely manner. Patient, during the quiet moments, should analyze and make an effort to remember all the follies that were committed and the resultant effects on the people who witnessed them. Most likely, such recollections will bring out the humor in the patient's mind which will prove to be a good release of blocked emotions, at the same time. Blocked emotions, and the constant effort to block them cost body energy which is in short supply with the patient. Patient should share such difficult but humorous experiences with his or her friends and intelligent relatives. This process is not only an acceptance of stroke occurrence, but also self induced therapy which is far better than outsourced therapy. Unless the patient accepts the stroke occurrence and the damage it has caused, it will be difficult to make a timely recovery. Although a lot of professionals believe that the patient can completely recover from a stroke occurrence after a period of time, but I as a non professional do not believe this assertion. In my opinion, once the damage is done, the patient can be cured to continue the daily life, however, all the damage is never cured completely. With continuous effort, the brain creates new areas of memory storage, and the process is slow and requires strengthening which takes many years of learning and practice. Even after relearning of all the lost memories and functions, prominent symptoms of stroke aftermath can suddenly reappear if drop in the energy level or excessive emotional stress is experienced. Therefore, stroke patient has got to be careful for the rest of life after the first stroke occurrence, otherwise, second, third and even fourth stroke will be repeated, that is if the patient is lucky to survive. The severity of such a repeated experience can be accumulative and will not be pleasant. Learn everything about stroke and heart disease, and avoid the first and the second experience.

AGING: Aging is a natural process for all plants, and life forms, including humans, which takes us to the ultimate pinnacle of maturity after which we cease to live. Aging is a process which reduces the degree of function that each organ, each gland, heart, brain, and all other parts of our body. It is common for people to experience with varied degrees the slowing down of the digestive system as people progress in years of life. For various reasons associated with aging people do not eat as much they used to do when they were young, primarily because the function of their digestive system has been reduced. Metabolizing capability of the body is reduced. Also, body does not produce all the enzymes and their required quantities that are needed for a healthy metabolism. This very trait compels us to eat smaller portions of food as we age. Acceptance of the fact that we are getting old will only lead to be at peace with ourselves and the natural phenomena, thereby the thought of aging does not become a burden on our mind, but instead it becomes a relief. Once it is established in the patient's mind that there will be a time in the future when the patient has to leave this known world, possessions, loved ones and friends; it will become increasingly easy and comfortable to do the right things to get better, appropriate and joyful social interactions, awareness of self and others in the process of living life, and the confidence to carry out daily chores whatever they happen to be. We will talk about a bit later about the ways to slow down, to a limited extend, the aging process of our body.

SOCIAL setting: Happy and congenial social environment is of high priority for all of us for a healthful life, and is very important for the stroke patients. People of all ages should be available to interact, and gestures of acceptance and accommodation from the people around will be highly therapeutic and beneficial for the patient. To have such a setting, the patient will have to move out of the hospital or care facility, or the confinement of home. Quite often, patients are left alone in the house, or with someone with whom the patient has no communication whatsoever. This is absolutely not good for the patient. Caregivers, or care attendants, or relatives should take the patient, if the patient is unable to manage to go alone, by himself or herself, to a public place like a community center, public part, or library, or a shopping mall, etc. where a lot of people of all ages and walks of life happen to be present. Patient will benefit from such a daily activity, because it will provide the patient a variety of instant associations with a vast number of experiences which were lost due to stroke. Such visitations will speed up the recollections and memory redevelopment. It will also amuse the patient who will feel happy and will look forward to the next visit. These are simple sources of satisfying experiences but very important and educational ones, because the patient is unable to participate in other worldly activities for some time to come. The motto should be to provide the patient all the good things in life which the patient can currently handle without aggravation and stress. Here we should remember that patient should make attempts to participate in the social system within the parameters of his or her current capabilities. While never stopping to carry out the participatory attempts, the patient should progress toward increased social interaction. Why? If the patient is absent from the social environment and exchanges for any length of time, then it may become much more difficult to re-enter the social scene at a later date. Patient could be left behind in the fast paced flow of life which the loved ones, friends, business associates, etc. are experiencing. It will be like returning to your home town after absence of 10 years and finding a complete change of social and business scene, and no one to say hello to. Therefore, social participation and its continuity are essential to patient's well being.

GEOGRAPHICAL location does play an important role in the patient's well being. Weather, terrain, altitude, etc. all play a significant part to determine the chances and the speed of patient's improvement. Patient needs interaction, outings, exercise, social setting, medical care, food shelter, etc. Those patients who can afford to move to a milder climate, they should, because it will provide them more opportunities to go out in public for educational, social, memory development, activity, and comfort reasons. Besides, warm weather is good for adequate blood circulation which the stroke and heart patients value. Cold weather does pose restrictions, and the patient may take much longer to recuperate from various disabilities. Small towns do not necessarily represent dull life. In face, some small towns provide more congenial and civilized opportunities for amusing social interactions than the big cities. Comfort for the patient, within the financial restraints, should be taken in to consideration at all times. If the patient can manage on his/her own with the help of loved ones or trusted relative, then efforts should be made to relocate in to a town of patient's choice.

ENVIRONMENT: Just stay away from noisy and irritating conditions; live in an environment with minimum pollution of air, water, chemicals, toxins, and electro magnetic pollution. Metals and toxic chemicals in the air, water, and the soil get in to our body, and cause havoc with our health and longevity. Some of these pollutants cause stroke and heart disease. Stroke and heart patients must make an effort to relocate to a cleaner environment. We know that heavy metals in the environment get in to our drinking water, foods, and air, and from there they get in to our body. These heavy metals can cause lesions in the walls of the blood vessels, which gives rise to blood clotting and in a short span of time blocking the artery. Blocked arteries block the blood flow to the brain, and brain cells die without the blood supply. Stroke patient has already experienced this life threatening condition which should not have to be repeated. Such an environment will be hazardous for the stroke patient no matter how great the medical help is available there.

CHOLESTEROL

Controlling High Cholesterol: diet, exercise, medication, and medical attention are some of the pre-requisites for controlling high cholesterol levels in the blood stream. Avoid animal fats, cholesterol containing foods, Trans fatty acids, stress, anger, etc. and try to learn eating vegetarian foods more often.

GENETICS: genes do play a predetermined role of high or low levels of cholesterols in our bodies, and for now only medication seems to be the solution besides other precautions. Incorporating vegetarian foods, avoiding fats, exercising, healthy social life, healthy geographical environment, peaceful and philosophical state of mind, meditation, etc. can beat the genetic odds for several years.

Over 80% of the people did not have high cholesterol under control in 2002, over 1.7 million Americans were told they had Cholesterol of 200mg/dl or higher. Just 10% decrease in the Cholesterol levels can significantly reduce the occurrence of Stroke or Heart Attack.

More than ½ of Americans do not know the Symptoms of a Stroke; only 17% of the people know the Symptoms of Stroke to call 911.

In general, Life Expectancy of Whites is higher than Blacks by 27%, and 8% due to Stroke. It says something; only 18% of Latin Americans have their Blood Pressure under control. Just for your information and the scope of this issue of Stroke, please consider the following mentioned:

Over 71 million American Adults are endowed with one or more types of Cardio Vascular Disease (CVD), and out of this number more than 27 million are 65 years or over. We all can assess the risk factors and eventualities. 65 million Americans have Systolic Pressure of Blood at 140mm/HG or greater, and Diastolic Pressure of Blood at 90mm/HG or greater, who happen to be under medication, or who have been advised at least twice about their High Blood Pressure (HBP) by their Physicians. On daily basis, loss of life due to Cardio Vascular Disease in America is very high. If we succeed in eliminating all forms of Cardio Vascular Disease, then life expectancy could go up to 84.6 years or more from 77.6 years.

ABOUT CHOLESTEROL:

Cholesterol is a soft and waxy substance found among the Lipids (FATS) in the blood stream and all body cells. It is an important part of a HEALTHY BODY. Our bodies use Cholesterol to form membranes of all cells, and also some of the hormones besides other functions

Our bodies have assigned special carriers to transport Cholesterol to and from the body cells. Strangely, Cholesterol and other fats cannot be dissolved in the blood, and therefore either they travel in the blood stream or get stuck and lodged in the walls of arteries. Mainly, there are two kinds of Lipoproteins:
Low Density Lipoproteins (LDL), and
High Density Lipoproteins (HDL)

LDL is the major Cholesterol Carrier in the blood. If too much LDL Cholesterol circulates in the blood, it can slowly build up in the walls of arteries feeding the heart and the Brain. LDL in large quantities in the blood stream can join other substances in the blood stream, thereby forming PLAQUE which is a thick and hard deposit in the walls of arteries.

PLAQUE can block arteries. This condition is called ATHEROSCLERO-SIS. A clot that is formed near the PLAQUE is called THROMBOSIS, which can cause a HEART ATTACK by causing blockage to the heart, or a BRAIN ATTACK by causing blockage of blood flow to the brain. LDL is the Bad Cholesterol, and should be less than 100mg/dl. Lower level of LDL Cholesterol is better, and reflects a lower risk of Heart Attack and Stroke.

HDL carries about one third of the Blood Cholesterol in our bodies. Medical experts think that HDL tends to carry Cholesterol away from the arteries, and bring back to the liver where it is passed through the body. While, other Medical experts believe that HDL removes excess Cholesterol from the PLAQUE and slows down their growth. HDL seems to protect our bodies from Stroke and Heart Attacks. HDL is the good Cholesterol. High HDL level is good for our body, because it takes some of LDL cholesterol and carries it to the liver for disposal. Also HDL blocks LDL and white blood cells to enter in to the arterials walls. HDL reduces the clotting of blood besides partially acting like an Antioxidant thereby stopping the oxidation of LDL in the blood stream. We enter a high risk zone when our HDL is

Less than 40mg/dl for Men

Less than 50mg/dl for Women

Therefore low HDL levels in our body are definitely a High Risk factor for us

LP class (a) Cholesterol is genetic variation of plasma LDL. High levels of LP class(a) Cholesterol is important risk factor for developing Atherosclerosis prematurely. Lesions in the walls of arteries contain substances that may interact with LP class (a) which stimulate building up of fatty deposits.

Our body produces 1000mgs of Cholesterol each and every day, so why to add additional Cholesterol. We do not need it at all, but we cannot avoid it under the current life style. It is recommended that we should take less than 300 mgs of cholesterol intake per day from the food source is recommended for those who do not suffer from heart or stroke condition. Less than 200 mgs of cholesterol per day from the food source is recommended for Stroke and Heart patients. Tobacco smoke lowers HDL (the good cholesterol) levels, and also it increases tendency for the blood to clot. Therefore, tobacco smoking is extremely hazardous for Stroke and Heart patients. Alcohol increases HDL (the good cholesterol) levels in the body, but in moderation only.

SOURCES OF CHOLESTEROL IN OUR FOOD

All animal products have cholesterol. Some of them are: eggs, beef, chicken, pork, shrimp, etc., and the foods that have high saturated fats or Trans fatty acids like: grilled cheese sandwiches, margarine, chicken salad, etc.

Cholesterol from foods enters your digestive track, and then it reaches your liver, and from there it can easily circulate throughout our bodies via our blood stream.

Also, our bodies produce cholesterol naturally, and our family history, Genes, play a significant role in this process. Most of the cholesterol in the blood stream comes from our own bodies. Throughout our bodies, the liver and other body cells make Cholesterol, and of course, this very cholesterol is circulated throughout our bodies via blood stream. When our intake of foods that are high in cholesterol is added to the cholesterol which our bodies have already produced, the result is high cholesterol. So. In other words, we are adding additional cholesterol (taken from the food source) to already well supplied cholesterol produced by our bodies. This results in the excess of cholesterol in our bodies.

Muscle weakness or any other weakness that cannot be explained must be attended to immediately, as this could be the result of High Cholesterol levels and possibly some blockage in the flow of blood at the location of weakness or pain.

ARRHYTHMIA is a source of Strokes and Heart Attacks, and occurs when the heart beat is too slow or too fast. Heart beat of 60 beats per minute is too slow, and 100 beats per minute is too fast. Or, the electrical impulses in the brain travel in abnormal pathways. All are danger to our well being. Primarily, the signals for danger are when heart beats are slow or fast, short or long, regular or irregular, light headedness, dizzy, faint, or even loss of consciousness, shortness of breath, unusual sensation, and palpitation. Palpitation can happen when we are at rest, or during a strenuous exercise. Palpitation starts suddenly or gradually.

PLAQUE

Plaque is a combination of cholesterol, other fatty substances, calcium, and blood components, and this combination of components stick together to the artery wall lining. Over a period of time, a hard shell forms and covers the plaque. Plaques have various sizes and shapes. There are hard and somewhat softer Plaques. The unstable and softer Plaques can rupture or burst open, thereby causing blood clotting inside the artery. If the blood clot ends up blocking the artery completely, it can stop the flow of blood completely resulting in Stroke or Heart Attack.

ARTERIOSCLEROSIS is also known as hardening of arteries. Arteries have several inner walls, and when the first, middle, and the inner walls lose elasticity and become harder due to accumulation of calcium and substances build up. Hardening of the arteries is one of the major causes of stroke and heart disease.

ATHEROSCLEROSIS is one of the types of arteriosclerosis, and represent a condition of clogged arteries as a result of plaque build up on the inside of the arterial walls. Cholesterol in the blood, damage to the artery wall, inflammation, etc. play important role in Plaque build up.

Researchers are studying how the Plaque actually develops and changes over time, how the arteries become damaged, and why Plaque can burst and break open giving way to blood clot formation. Although the exact causes are not definable, but there are some indicators which are directly related to it. The important indicators are: high blood cholesterol, over weight, smoke from tobacco. lack of exercise, lethargic life style, high blood pressure, stressful life, and some other factors.

The recommended preventive measure would include:

Maintaining appropriate body weight levels

Get plenty of regular exercise which you can maintain for the rest of your life

Healthy diet: (low saturated fats), intake of plentiful vegetables, fruits, etc.

Get the High Blood Pressure and High Cholesterol treated by a Physician

If you have Diabetes, then get treated by a Physician

If you smoke, then stop smoking

Reduce stress by various methods as suggested in this book and otherwise.

HYPERTENSION is often described as the Silent Killer. It is caused by:

Anxiety caused by various life circumstances

Sustained high stress levels constrict the arteries resulting in restricted blood flow

Pressure in the arteries buids up, slowly or rapidly

Heart happens to be working harder than normal

Constricted blood vessels are holding back the flow of blood

Consistent levels of high blood pressure

Extra wear and tear of blood vessels, resulting in certain areas to weaken,

And these weakened areas can become the cause of Stroke and Heart Attack.

AGE FACTOR

Ageing is a natural process

Arteries become fragile with age

Arteries become less elastic, less flexible, and become hardened

Hardened and less elastic arteries slow down the normal flow of blood

Lack of elasticity and flexibility in the hardened arteries with below normal flow of blood cause arteries to get clogged

Stroke or heart attack will become of high probability

DIABETES

Diabetics are three times more likely to have a storke or heart attack

They are twice more likely to have hypertension

42% Stroke and heart patients also have diabetes

Diabetics are more prone to high cholesterol, and obesity.

FAMILY HISTORY

We all know now that Genes play the most important role in our lives. Somehow, genes create a Physical Destiny in our lives, and it seems that we are captive to this design of nature. If we carry a family history of Cardio Vascular Disease, (CVD), or High Blood Pressure (HBP), then the probability is very high of experiencing physical damage from these diseases. By proper precautions and medication, we can delay such occurrences for several years at least, if not for decades.

CHOLESTEROL LEVELS

Above 100mg/dl of LDL will take you to the Risk Zone

Lower than 50mg/dl of HDL will take Men to the Risk Zone, and

Lower than 60 mg/dl of HDL will take Women to the Risk Zone.

Dr. Bob Arnot has developed several formulas within the field of stroke and heart attack conditions. According to him the safe limits for cholesterol in the body are:

Total cholesterol count should be less than 200

LDL should be less than 100 mg/dl

HDL should be more than 60 mg/dl

TOBACCO

Tobacco smoking lowers the HDL levels in the body, Increases the tendency for the Blood to clot. Nicotine and carbon monoxide reduces the oxygen in blood, also, they damage the walls of blood vessels, thereby creating a situation for clots to form. Birth control pills and smoking increase the chances of having a stroke or heart attack. Smoking tobacco provides the smoker a supply of about 4,000 compounds of chemicals, and is the leading cause of stroke/heart disease. It damages the coronary arteries, harms the aorta, and causes sudden brain/heart attacks. Smoking provides adequate supply of nicotine, nitrosamine, tar, pesticides, carbon monoxide, volatile organic compounds, (benzene), cadmium (metal), radio active polonium (metal), carbonyl compounds, polycyclic aromatic hydro carbons, etc. There are about 400 carbon compounds in tobacco smoking that are lethal to humans. First and second hand tobacco smoke is most dangerous to humans, and can be the cause of stroke or heart attack.

VARICOSE VEINS: varicose veins appear on legs when the valves in the veins do not function properly. In healthy veins, several valves keep the blood moving toward the heart. This blood is on the return journey to the heart after completing its route to nourish various parts of the body and the legs. Heart sends out oxygen rich blood to various parts of the body via the arteries, and the used up and oxygen poor blood is returned to the heart via the veins. The oxygen in returning blood which is contained in the veins has been used up. There are several valves in the veins which help the blood to rise and reach to the heart. When these valves become weak and stop functioning properly, the blood does not rise to the heart. The blood remains in the leg veins and becomes stagnant which causes the veins to swell or become large and visible.

Defective valves in the veins are caused by too much standing in one place, or too much sitting in one position, crossing the legs for a long period of time, increased pressure in the abdomen, or insufficient activity, etc. Often pregnant women suffer from varicose veins due to increase pressure in the abdomen and insufficient activity. Varicose veins can result in pain in the leg, cramps, skin ulcers near the ankles, skin around ankles change its color to brown, swelling of ankles, heaviness and fullness in the leg, legs feel heavy or loaded, visible enlarged veins, etc. Such symptoms of varicose veins should not be ignored because they can prove to be of great danger to all, but especially to stroke and heart patients, or to a potential stroke or heart patient. If unattended, varicose veins can cause Deep Vein Thrombosis (DVT) which can lead to Pulmonary Embolism. Pulmonary Embolism is when a blood clot from any part of the body, in this case from varicose veins, breaks free and travels toward the lung, heart, or brain. Often, such symptoms appear in people who drive for a long distance without taking breaks, travelers in the economy class on a long flight, sick and hospitalized patients, It is also linked to genes with the blood clot abnormalities, and cancer. Patients who come out of surgery of knee, hip, chest, calf, stomach, etc. can also become candidates for developing blood clot which can travel toward the lung, heart, or brain. Also, leg cramps are closely associated with DVT, Recently, David Bloom, NBC reporter covering Iraq war, died suddenly. The reported cause of his sudden death was due to a blood clot that formed in his leg, which traveled up to his lungs where it blocked the flow of blood. He died of it. This is typical example of Pulmonary Embolism which is generally caused by sitting for a long time in a small and tight space like sitting in an economy class seat on a commercial flight. He had been complaining about pain in his leg and could not pinpoint the reason for it. Also, it is possible that he suffered from dehydration from the desert heat which caused the depletion of minerals and thickened the blood. About 60.000 Americans die from this each year. Many researchers believe that it is genetic, and in some cases may be true, however, Dr. Gabe Mirkin, Diane Mirkin, and Dr. Paolo Prandoni of Italy think that it is caused by atherosclerosis or hardening of arteries.

Leg cramps are not uncommon among the general population. It is quite common for the stroke and heart patients to experience cramps in the calf and thigh. The pain emanating from the cramp may vary from slight to extremely painful. Also, this is similar to the pain which is experienced in the chest or just below the rib cage where heart is located, known as angina, heart attack or something like that. Cramp in the leg is caused by lack of minerals like sodium (salt), calcium, and magnesium, and a few other less known reasons. When these minerals get depleted we tend to get cramps. Depletion occurs when we exert our body to too much exercise, or heat by which we end up losing fluid from our body. Therefore, we need to drink extra quantities of water if we expose ourselves to heat and exercise. Malnutrition is another reason for having leg cramps. Lack of calcium, salt, and magnesium can result in getting cramps. Also, lack of blood circulation causes leg cramps, and that is why staying active is important for adequate circulation of blood. Severe leg cramps can occur due to inadequate flow of blood in the leg, which can be due to **Deep Vein Thrombosis** (DVT). If you are out in the heat or walking a long distance when you could bring out a sweat then do drink water, take calcium and magnesium containing foods. In the absence of all these, just put a half a pinch of salt in your water before drinking.

Although, varicose veins may be a common sight in every day life, but it should not be taken lightly. If you are a stroke or heart disease potential or a patient, then you must consult the doctor and work on the possibilities of curing the varicose veins condition. Chances of blood clot developing are very high among patients who have medical conditions like Stroke, Heart Disease, Inflammatory Bowel Disease, Pregnancy, etc. Breaking away blood clot and traveling toward lung, heart, and brain is also linked to women who take birth control pills. These symptoms appear in the legs of men and women who could suffer from the consequences of traveling blood clot. The medical community is finding similar blood clot breaking free from various locations in the upper body as well. It is common for the nurse to insert a long, thin, and flexible tube in the arm vein for various procedures. This process irritates the veins, and causes blood clot to form. Also, pace makers implanted in the patients' chest can cause blood clots to form. If there is a formation of cancer near the vein, then it will be a strong possibility for the blood clot to form. Although it is quite rare, but the possibility cannot be ignored of the fact that constant and repeated activity of a certain body limb can give way to blood clot formation. For example, baseball pitcher, weightlifting athlete, swimmers, etc. can suffer from the blood clot formation, which can travel to the lungs, heart and the brain. In general, the probability of developing Deep Vein Thrombosis is high among over weight and obese people, stroke and heart patients, pregnant women, nursing mothers, etc.

There are several treatments that are offered by the medical community to cure the Varicose Veins in the legs. One is to remove these enlarged veins from the legs by surgery. Doctor can prescribe an anticoagulant or blood thinner which decreases the chances for the blood to clot. Also, through laser the doctor can seal the enlarged vein, and have the blood routed via alternative route. For knowledge, do check with the society for vascular surgery of Chicago, IL at vascular@vascularsociety.org, and Sims, Inc. of Colierville, TN at info@stopvaricoseveins.com.

I suggest that Varicose Veins can be treated by your own self without taking any medication, or surgical procedures. I have had varicose veins, both on the side and the calf area of my left leg for about 25 years. In addition to that there is some brown colored skin just above the inside of my left ankle. I have been able to reduce the swelling, as well as the discoloration to a great extent. I still have some visible varicose veins and some discoloration remaining on my left leg, primarily because of my lack of consistent discipline to adhere to my chosen diet and regular walking. I get side tracked with good food and laziness from time to time. However, when I do adhere to the right diet and sufficient walking on daily basis in a consistent manner, then I do notice a complete disappearance of varicose veins on my left leg, and also I notice that the discoloration just above my left ankle becomes minimal and hardly visible. My experience may be a bit different than what your doctor would recommend you to do. Nevertheless, do try this because this method would not only reduce ugly sight of varicose veins and the danger they pose to you, but also would prove to be beneficial for your overall physical and mental health. You do not need to spend extra money to do this.

If you can walk, then walk daily for at least half an hour, and if you can do more then so much the better, because walking exercise can be consistently maintained most of the span of life. When you are in your house, apartment, or room, keep your legs moving. For example, pace the floor while you are watching TV, or doing something else which does not require sitting. Just keep your legs and feet moving as much as you can manage to do so. When you have to sit, then try to lift your legs up whenever it is convenient to do so. Do not cross your legs while in a sitting position, instead leave them independent of each other. Some people say cross them at the ankles, but I suggest that each leg should be kept separate from the other in a sitting position. Like, while sitting on a chair and putting your feat on the corner of the table just in front of you will do wonders for your legs. It will be even better if your chair is lower than the table you wish to rest your feat. Your elevated feat will send the blood toward your upper body and the heart, which is good for you because then the heart can reprocess this oxygen poor blood once again. Intermittently, raise your feet up for a few minutes whenever you find it comfortable to do so throughout the day. There is another very important thing that I learned and practiced to make the varicose veins disappear from my leg has been maintaining a very clean stomach. I found that there was a direct relationship between the state of my stomach and the enlargement of the varicose veins. The day my stomach is clean, and my diet is vegetarian, without too much of sugar, fats and salt, in just adequate quantity with enough water, the varicose veins disappear or they are barely visible. Also, I found that using fresh lemon or lime juice in your salads or in your meals does help to reduce the varicose veins. Each time I notice some improvement, I go out for a walk, because it provides me with opportunity to capitalize on the satisfactory health condition, and make it even better. Consumption of vegetables, grains, fat free yogurt, little cheese, fat free milk, sugars from fruits only, no fats, very little salt, and a lot of water helped me to keep my stomach and the blood clean. Therefore, walking, lifting your feet and legs up, keeping your stomach clean, and the right diet can make the varicose veins disappear, as it is experienced by me when I am maintaining discipline.

CHAPTER IV

DURING AND AFTER STROKE AND HEART DISEASE

Often, it is very difficult for the patient to determine if the stroke is occurring, or it has already occurred. But with understanding the usual symptoms of stroke, any one can know if a stroke occurrence is imminent, or if a stroke has already occurred. The pain in the head, a crucifying headache, seems to be constant before and after the Stroke. The following mentioned are most commonly experienced after the Stroke, and its realization:

Mood swings for no apparent reason is quite a common occurrence after the Stroke. Emotional Liability is another name for it. Uncontrollable crying, or laughing, depression, various disabilities, loss of friends, loss of vocation etc are common aftermaths of stroke

Ironically, the patient is not completely aware of the injuries to his or her body, and he or she tends to carry on with life as if everything is as before. Typically, the patient becomes unaware of the fact that he or she has not completed a specific task, but believes that it has been completed. Like not dressing completely, or shaving one side of the face, and thinking that the task has been completed. Bumping in to the furniture, driving through the red light, ignoring the affected limbs' incapability, etc. are just a few examples of such conditions.

Patient cannot seem to recognize and understand the every day familiar objects the way they were perceived before. Objects may seem nearer or farther than they actually are. For example, spilling coffee at the table, not making an accurate contact between the spoon full of food and the mouth, colliding with people while walking, knocking the hand with the corner of cabinet while taking some object out of it, falling from the steps, bath, or toilet, inability to stay on the sidewalk, inability to walk in a straight line, etc are some of the common occurrences.

There is a remarkable affect on the stroke patient's vision. If it is not temporarily lost for a short period of time, it is definitely reduced to a significant degree. Not understanding speech and difficulty in saying the things patient is actually thinking to say is called **APHASIA**. Inability to talk, listen, read and write is very common among the stroke patients.

Tongue, lips, palate muscles become weak, and speech becomes slow, slurred or distorted (called **DYSARTHRIA**). People cannot understand what the patient is saying

Ability to think clearly disappears. Patient thinks of doing something at the table, but upon reaching that table patient cannot recall the reason of his arrival there. The patient may decide to go to the kitchen to have a glass of water, but once in the kitchen the patient may not remember the purpose of his or her being there, even if the patient looks at the glass itself. Short term memory gets lost. It may take several minutes or even much longer to realize the purpose.

There are some commonly associated affects of Stroke and its location of occurrence in the brain:

If the Stroke occurred in the Right Brain, then the left side will be affected.

- Numbness and weakness on the left side of the body
- Difficulty in performing even simple daily tasks
- Perception difficulties
- Disorientation of time, day, month
- Loss of left vision field
- Visual memory loss
- Abstract thinking will become almost impossible
- Very short attention span, with almost no focus capabilities
- Lack of energy, resulting in lethargy
- Intense emotions with highs and lows
- Poor or lack of judgment
- Impulsiveness and unconventional behavior

If the Stroke occurred in the Left Brain, the right side will be affected

- Numbness and weakness of the right side of the body
- Partial or complete loss of speech
- Partial or complete loss of understanding your own language
- Difficulty or complete loss of comprehension of written text and spoken word
- Inability to see errors, and very poor judgment
- Confusion between left and right
- Loss of visual field on the right,
- Significantly decreased memory
- Slowness in all actions

- Loss of energy

- Helplessness and depression

HYPERTENSION is very common condition after the Stroke, it can linger on for quite a long time. Elevated Blood Pressure and highly tense state is experienced. Patient will be on the edge most of time, will be agitated, and will not hesitate to pick a fight, or demonstrate disagreement. Problem is aggravated when after the stroke, lower Blood Pressure may not supply the blood to the areas that have already been affected by the blood supply blockage. In other words, blood supply does not reach adequately to the affected area which caused the Stroke. But body naturally tries to supply blood to all parts of the body, even if it is affected by an injury. Unfortunately, this process makes the Blood Pressure to rise which, in turn, is dangerous for the patient. A lot of opinions about this exist, and simultaneously a lot of research is being carried out to find a suitable and therapeutic solution to this problem. In my opinion the best solution is that the patient should remove himself or herself from the scene that stimulates aggression, pugnacity, excitement, and hypertension right away.

DIABETICS face a serious dilemma after suffering from a Stroke. Body's response to the trauma and physical stress of Stroke often includes a boost in the Blood Sugar of the patient, whether the patient is Normal or Diabetic. Also, after the Stroke, a combination of medical problems occur due to restricted levels of activities, and diet change which adversely affects the Sugar Levels in the body—especially affecting the persons with Diabetes. Patients with or without Diabetes must be monitored for Sugar Levels to remain under control, or within the acceptable levels. The best would be that patient initiates periodic glucose tests voluntarily by making it a routine. In this way, the patient will feel responsible and in control.

There have been several physical ailments I went through, and I thought that were only happening to me. But after reading Dr. Joel Stern's impressive writings I was convinced that it was common for stroke and heart patients to experience such disabilities. Dr. Stern has described several health problems as if he was transcribing my experiences. In the following lines you will find his descriptions bearing complete similarities to some of my experiences.

BLADDER problems are very common among stroke and heart patients. Stroke and heart attack often affects the bladder function in the body. Inability to pass urine even if the Bladder is full is caused by the temporary weakness of the muscle in the Bladder. This bladder muscle squeezes the urine out. Also, the patient's mind fails to read the signal that it is time to empty the full Bladder. Urinary Incontinence occurs and patients lose control over emptying of Bladder. It becomes involuntary on the patients part. It is a common problem after the Stroke. Patients experiencing **URINARY INCONTINENCE** have another predicament to deal with., and that is after the Stroke patient's mind becomes so confused, and either they are unable to reach the "decision level" to empty the Bladder, or they do not know how to communicate their such needs to the Care-Giver, because Patient's mind is impaired, speech is impaired, memory is lost, etc. Care-Givers must be trained to understand and anticipate Patient's needs under such MULTIMPLE LEVELS of DISABLED condition. Often, URINARY INFECTION is the outcome of INCONTINENCE. Medical help should be the obvious approach to combat this condition.

However, I do suggest an exercise which may help the patient to control incontinence. The exercise involves squeezing the pelvic muscle and then releasing it after a few seconds. How to find the pelvic muscle? At the time of urinating, concentrate hard and then stop urinating just in the middle of it. At first it will be a bit difficult, so try a couple of times. If the patient succeeds in stopping the urine just for 5 to 10 seconds, the patients will feel some pressure in the lower part of the belly. That point where the pressure from stopping the urine is felt should be remembered. That point is the pelvic muscle. Now the identification of pelvic muscle has been made, the exercise comes next. In the privacy of your room, standing, or sitting, you can squeeze the same part of the body, the pelvic muscle, and release it after a few seconds. Do this exercise a few times, whenever it is convenient for you. If possible combine this exercise with stomach squeezing exercises. You will be surprised that you have accomplished something important, and you will be able to control the time to visit the bathroom for urination.

URINARY INFECTION is something probable in Stroke and heart patients, and cannot be ignored, or minimized. Urinary retention causes INFECTION. Inability to urinate, or not recognizing the need to urinate, results in urine to stagnate in the Bladder, which allows Bacteria to get established in the Bladder and the Urinary Track.

FREQUENT URINATION is also experienced by some Stroke and Heart patients, even in the absence of urine infection. Patients may feel frequent urge to urinate in spite of the fact that their Bladder may be empty. This is because the Patient almost loses control over the muscle controlling the Bladder. This muscle which controls the Bladder is called DETRUSSOR MUSCLE. In some patients, this Detrussor Muscle becomes over active and the patients feel the urge to urinate. Stomach and pelvic muscle exercises will reduce this uncomfortable health condition.

BOWEL MOVEMENT PROBLEMS are very common among patients after the Stroke or Heart attack. After the stroke or heart attack, constipation sets in primarily due to immobility, changes in diet, inadequate liquid intake, cognitive and communication issues, impaired body apparatus, low energy, lethargy, inability to empty the stomach, etc. Dietary fiber and a lot of liquids must be put on diet. Care-Givers should be trained to know such crucial needs of patients. A lot of fiber is healthy for all of us, but it will prove to be very unhealthy if it is not combined with sufficient liquids, preferably water. Fiber without liquids in the body can cause severe constipation, which causes a host of ailments entirely separate from stroke and heart conditions.

SEIZURES are uncontrolled ELECTRICAL activity in the brain that results in loss of consciousness, uncontrolled body movements (shaking & shivering). Damage in the left brain from a Stroke can cause a SCAR to form in the brain which then creates conditions for an uncontrolled Electrical activity. SEIZURE starts. The Seizure which affects just a part of the brain is called FOCUL, and an uncontrolled twitching of a body part is experienced by the patient. If FOCUL spreads to other parts of the brain, then it is called GENERALIZED SEIZURE which results in loss of consciousness.

HYDROCEPHALUS is a known condition which is caused by stroke. Brain is surrounded and protected by a clear protective fluid known as CEREBRO SPINAL FLUID (CSF). This fluid is produced inside the cavities of Middle Brain, known as VENTRICLES. If Stroke occurs in this vicinity of the brain, the flow of CSF can be blocked. The blocked fluid can build up inside the brain, causing a condition known as HYDRO-CEPHALUS. This blockage resulted from Stroke can cause DEATH. In less severe cases, confusion, incontinence, gradual neurological deterioration are very common.

VENOUS THROMBOSIS is a condition to which Stroke or heart patient is pre-disposed to, primarily due to reduced physical activity as a result of stroke or heart attack. Patients develop Blood Clots in the legs, known as DEEP VENOUS THROMBOSIS (DVT). This condition can occur even in people who do not have stroke or heart disease history, however, it can lead to them. These clots are of Life Threatening potential. If these Blood Clots are dislodged, they can travel to the Lungs, a life threatening condition known as PULMONARY EMBOLISM. The best treatment for this is first preventing DVT and then Pulmonary Embolism.

OSTEOPOROSIS & FRACTURES are thinning of bones, or loss of bones that lead to fractures. Although it is associated with the disease of OLDER WOMEN, it is common for Stroke and heart patients to suffer from it. Almost all the old people suffer from this disease in some degree, however, in Stroke patients it affects the LIMBS and BODY PARTS that were affected by the Stroke. For Stroke patients, falls and fractures can prove to be extremely dangerous. Regular exercise, bearing weights around the ankles and walking with them are some of the important recommendations for Stroke patients. I was never diagnosed for osteoporosis, but after taking the ultra sound scanning test which I took voluntarily, outside my health insurance coverage, it was revealed that I was beginning to have this condition. This report explained the cause of some consistent pain in my heels, and loss of some bone in my teeth.

EDEMA is swelling of various body parts and limbs. After the stroke or heart attack, reduced movement, lack of exercise and activity often leads to EDEMA (SWELLING) of the affected limbs and body parts. There is always a tendency on the part of patients to avoid using the affected limb or body parts, thereby resulting in lack of normal pumping action which happens with the movements, and helps to remove the liquid from the effected limb or body part. EDEMA may be the crucial sign of formation of BLOOD CLOT in the leg (DEEP VENOUS THROMBOSIS). If actual exercise and walking are not possible for a stroke or heart patient, then regular raising and lowering the effected limb would create a pumping action by increasing and decreasing the blood circulation by such movements.

PNEUMONIA often complicates the survival and recovery of Stroke and Heart patients. Although it is less common to happen, precautionary measures are vitally important.

SLEEP DISTURBANCE & DISORDER is common among Stroke patients primarily because of confusion, disorientation, movement difficulties, etc. Total mental function is affected by Stroke, and there goes the sleep cycles, mental clock, sleep rhythm.

SLEEP APNEA is the failure to breath during sleep. Body's protection system wakes up the patient when breathing is blocked. SNORING is one of the signs of Sleep Apnea.

FATIGUE & LACK OF ENERGY is probably the most common conditions experienced after the stroke or heart attack.Regular rest periods and naps become necessary, quite often just after performing a small tasks like brushing the teeth, making coffee, etc.

ARTERIOSCLEROSIS

Arteries have several layers of walls within. Healthy arteries are elastic and flexible. When the first layer, then the middle layer, and later the inner layers start to lose elasticity and get calcified, this change is called degenerative. It is commonly called: HARDENING OF ARTERIES. It is strongly believed that the origin of this degenerative change is DIABETIC condition.

ATHEROSCLEROSIS is one of several kinds of ARTERIOSCLEROSIS. It is a degenerative change in the walls of arteries, primarily the larger ones which are AORTA, CORONARY, AND CEREBRAL vessels. This degenerative change causes NARROWING OF ARTERIES. This narrowing process is caused by PLAQUE formation on the inner walls of the Blood Vessels, which causes the narrowing of arteries.

Also, ATHEROSCLEROSIS (narrowing of arteries) causes EMBOLISM. Embolism occurs when a piece of PLAQUE breaks away and gets in to the blood circulation thereby producing disastrous consequences. 70% to 80% of Plaque is tissue, Cholesterol, and other Fats. When Plaque breaks away and gets in to the blood stream, it can cause rupture of inner wall of artery. Rupture of inner wall of artery causes blood clots to take formation, through natural response of the body, which can partially or totally block the artery, and cause stroke or heart attack. If the break away piece of Plaque partially or totally blocks the artery, the result will be a definite stroke or heart attack.

ARTHRITIS will appear in almost every bone joint of the body resulting in a feeling of lifelessness. Patients will experience absence of energy and strength. Arthritis is not only debilitating but it can be extremely painful, and can stop the patient from doing anything. This fear of pain may get associated with most movements of the body.

It is always good to know at least something about the Stroke and Heart Attack. The probability of having a stroke or heart attack is so high in the United States, that is, if you have crossed the age of 50, then it is a must-to-know subject, and without some knowledge of it, one could classify this lack of knowledge to be ACHYLE'S HEEL. I know this first hand, because I went through this several times. The first 3 times were the most difficult. My anger toward certain people and my ignorance brought me to the experience of Stroke, but my determination to face the challenge and the pure natural instinct to survive saved me, at least for now.

Mayo Clinic has been actively involved in research on many diseases and Cardio Vascular Disease is among them. According to Mayo Clinic, Atherosclerosis will eventually develop in almost everybody as we grow old. Aging reduces elasticity in the body and the arteries, which causes muscles cells to degenerate. Degenerated muscles cells are partially replaced by fibrous tissues. The lining in the arteries gets weakened and damaged causing blood platelets to stick to the site of damage or injury. This triggers cholesterol and other substance like calcium to build up inside the arterial wall. Plaque is formed

CHAPTER V

BASIC RECOMMENDATIONS & THERAPIES

Even though my will to survive and get better was at all time high, I was continuously getting weaker, and in fact my several hour ordeal with my Healthcare Provider speeded up the process of big time weakness and loss of energy. The affect of stroke was taking place, and the general physical state seemed to be deteriorating. My lesson at this stage was: DO NOT HAVE LENGTHY CONVERSATION, DO NOT GET IN TO A SITUATION WHERE YOU ARE REQUIRED TO ANSWER MANY QUESTIONS REPEATEDLY. In subsequent years I learned that ARGUMENTS, DISCUSSIONS, and ANGER can almost KILL a stroke or heart patient within a short period of time. Stroke patient has lost MEMORY, or is gradually losing it as a result of stroke. Stroke patient finds it extremely difficult to remember things and words which are the constituents of making a conversation. Health providers, caregivers, loved ones, and friends end up asking too many questions whether to help the stroke patient, or just to demonstrate their love and sympathy, or just for curiosity. Additionally, these loved ones also contradict you in a small or significant way, which causes a lot of stress and anger in the mind of Stroke patient who finds himself or herself completely helpless and frustrated. Imagine a beggar begging for a loaf of bread and the people respond "you look good, your cheeks are rosy", "you look healthy", "you don't need bread", or "you got to be kidding", etc..

All these medical professionals and genius level people do not make an attempt to understand the stroke patient's predicament due to deteriorating, or deteriorated speech capability, memory loss, general weakness, insecurity, frustration of not being understood, On top of this miserable state of stroke patient's condition, all these professionals and well wishers will have somewhat common response: "YOU LOOK GOOD", "THERE IS NOTHING WRONG WITH YOU", "GIVE ME A CALL SOME-TIME", to stroke patient's expectation of some HELP. Even though, these people witnessed the open wound on the side of my head (later in two other locations of my head), blurred eyes, verbal disability, walking difficulties, and a red rash around half of my neck on the left side during the first Stroke, they continued to create a distance between myself and their fortresses. I could never learn the reason for the appearance of wide red band encircled around the left side of my neck. I could not get any answers from my doctor either. I did spit blood every day for about 9 to 10 months, and I experienced swallowing difficulty and some roughness inside the left side of my throat. Slowly the blood blemish went away and I stopped spitting blood, swallowing food and liquids become less difficult. I believed that nothing could stop me from getting well and fit again. It is a long process of healing, and patience, discipline, and determination are required, which can be accomplished by taking charge of your own healing process.

The time period during, immediately after, and at least 3 months following the Stroke is absolutely critical, and the CARE, UNDERSTAND-ING, ACCOMMODATION, LOVE, QUIET AND PEACEFUL ATMOSPHERE, SINCERE CONSIDERATIONS.... will only determine the degree of DISABILITY and chances of SURVIVAL.. At this point, and perhaps all the time, that surviving a stroke is one thing and living a life with at least some enjoyment is another. No matter what the compiled statistical data has been accumulated over the years by various institutions and researchers, once a stroke is experienced, there is **NO COMPLETE RECOVERY**, no matter who it is and how fit and good looking that person might become after a stroke occurrence.

There is survival, but no complete recovery. Just in a few days after the Stroke, I had forgotten to walk, and I seemed determined to proceed in my own way which probably was deteriorating me and leading me deeper in to other health problems and disability, and eventually to the incidence of subsequent strokes. I was not stopping life because I had had a stroke even though I was partially disabled, and almost completely disabled in some other areas. To a much lesser degree, I still experience the common disability factors that affected me during various strokes. When I feel fatigued or am experiencing low energy levels, my legs, ankles, and feet feel and act differently. During those times, it seems that they have developed their own brain, or they are not in harmony with my brain. My walking standards very much resemble to my walking when I was 20 years old, which should be readjusted to my current age. After 10 to 15 minutes of walking, they come to walking rhythm. Quite often I have to slightly change the left toe's point of direction a bit toward inside, and after a few minutes it becomes normal. Also, I am still experiencing hitting the corners of tables, chairs, corners of the cabinets and drawers when I reach to get something from the inside, hitting my toes to the furniture, etc which I relate to low energy levels. But such incidents have decreased in numbers. I suggest that stroke and heart attack patients should wear shoes, possibly sneakers, all the time, which will help them to avoid any injuries to the toes. When we are weak and somewhat older healing of wounds, especially in the legs and feet, take much longer than it did when we were younger.

I remember that just after the first stroke, I could not see the images on my TV, it was too difficult to concentrate even to focus on a face, or a plant. Images appeared as blur of light for several days or weeks, and after focusing hard the outlines of faces and things appeared in the field of vision. It took me quite some time to reach the level of seeing something on TV. The next phase was to stay focused on the screen and try to understand what it was, and so on. It was a gradual process, step by step, to reach the next level of understanding the pictures on TV and then relating it to the sounds. Much later I realized that I had very little comprehension, and barely I could make out as to what was being said in relation to what was being shown. I felt fantastic after accomplishing this task which eventually became the most useful tool to read and understand English once again.

I needed a nap after every small activity, like: brushing teeth, shaving, shower, making coffee, drinking, putting on clothes, etc. Another interesting factor that was quite noticeable was that quite often I shaved one side of the face and left the other side unshaved without recognizing the difference. I had difficulty remembering the number of cups of water I had put in the coffee pot and I had to empty and refill the pot a couple of times each morning, because I could not retain the number of cups I already put in. After finishing the shave and shower ritual in the morning instead of wearing day clothes, sometime I used to get in my pajamas again and start making the bed again, and then catching up with my folly several minutes later. For several years, I used to prepare my bed to go to sleep just as soon as I returned from outside chores, often at 3–4 O' Clock in the afternoon. In other words, the activities, sequences, order and system went out of the brain operating system. During winter time, I walked out just in a shirt without the winter coat, and after 5 minutes being outside realized that I was uncomfortable due to some unknown reason but could not pin point it, and then the message of cold weather and associated chill used to enter my mind making me to return back to my apartment. Removing the clothes from washer or dryer was another chore. I used to keep looking in to these machines to see if any clothes were left there. Sometime, I had to repeat my visits to the laundry room just to make sure washer and dryer were completely empty. My eyes were looking at the empty machines, but the message was not reaching my brain, or my brain was not processing the information. There are a variety of examples when messages to the brain were delayed, or when the brain failed to process the information received, and the subsequent action was either not taken or delayed.

I used to watch a lady of about late 60s who was quite aggressive in getting better and it seemed that she was succeeding on her own. I never saw anyone with her ever. She was a stroke patient. She could not drive, so she used to walk to the grocery store almost every day, and bring back one bag of groceries with her. That was all she could manage to carry. Each time we ran in to each other, she would stop briefly to tell me: "I am very hungry, I am starving, I want a hot meal "Each time, very casually I directed her attention to the bag she was holding. She used to look at it and walk away with some niceties. At other times, I saw her rushing back to her apartment after reaching half way to the grocery store by commenting that she had left the kitchen stove on and there could be some fire. I was very much familiar with these scenarios because I was doing it myself. I still do it after so many years. Retaining a piece of information for longer than few minutes, sometime even for a fraction of a minute, becomes difficult.

After witnessing such situations, I used to experience a great amount of pity, and I used to find extremely difficult to pull myself out of such feelings. After stroke, women and men who happen to be by themselves without loved ones or caregivers are in very pitiable circumstances. Somehow, our social and medical systems are not designed to accommodate such people, at least not as yet. It is alright to receive sympathy and extend sympathy to others, but this does not help the patient to be in the community of patients with similar or different ailments. Stroke patient must have a variety of people under diverse conditions around whenever it is possible, because stroke patient is a small child who has to learn everything once again. The things the patient still can remember must be reinforced regularly and for which the patient has got to be exposed to average life experiences. It is like a crash course the patient has to complete. Physically, it happens to be equally difficult challenge. The structure remains the same, but the inside becomes lose and weak like that of a child.

The weakness becomes the foe. Just do not fight it, otherwise you will get hurt. As a result of stroke I experienced **ARTHRITIS** in almost every bone joint with weak tendons and ligaments, and with completely no strength. Arthritic pain is quite uncomfortable, especially when it is in every joint of the body. I had a strong grip and could open almost any jammed glass jar, but after the stroke I could not unscrew a soda bottle. I could not open a milk carton. For about 6 months or so I used to take a small kitchen knife and used to jab at the top of the carton, which used to create an opening in the carton. What a challenging and funny time it was. There was no time to get bored; I was busy all the time just handling very simple things all day. Almost anything I did was not without pain, especially in the bone joints. Don't hesitate to talk to your doctor on regular basis regarding your pain and weakness and especially arthritic condition. However, I will report to you the way I cured my arthritic condition, physical weakness, weak ligaments and tendons. I continuously forced myself to carry out the things I had to do. In my wrists, elbows, knuckles, knees, ankles, etc. there was enough pain on a daily basis. I punished myself by using them on a regular basis. This is the way; I cured my excruciating pain in the right elbow and right shoulder many years ago, may be 20 years before having stroke. Just a few years ago, I cured pain in my right knee, and now I can climb stairs without any difficulty. I read somewhere that antioxidants, vitamin C, and manganese have some curing affect on arthritis, so I found foods that contain this nutrition. So besides repeatedly using the pain giving joint, I consumed beans, nuts, oatmeal, oranges, spinach, raisins, and blue berries whenever I could manage to do so. I did not take any capsules or medication whatsoever, and eventually got better. I have never hesitated to recommend this method to anyone with arthritic pain. Your intake of Calcium must correspond to its usage, without fail. What cures one person may not cure another, so use your own judgment and effort to get better., because each one of us is different in the way of genes, age, height, weight, habits, foods, environment, race, lifestyles, etc.

Where I live now, I witness on daily basis at least a couple of neighbors, with a stroke history, doing things I know very well because I had done them in a similar manner, and sometime I still do. There is a gentleman who comes to pick up his mail from his mail box. He stands in front of his mail box and looks at it for several minutes, and then he puts his hand in pocket for the keys. He is still looking at the mail box. He takes the keys out and after fumbling a bit he inserts the key in lock and leaves it there. After a few minutes, he opens it and looks at the mail in the mail box for several minutes. He pulls the mail out of the box and looks at it again for several minutes, etc. He spends about 30 minutes in the whole exercise of picking up his mail. He waits a few minutes before he presses the elevator button. I admire these people who have the courage to overcome the disabilities after the stroke, and continue to improve.

There is a lady who I see often. She started to use a walker after the stroke, and now she walks every afternoon for quite some time. She had a stroke just a few days after her husband was taken by an ambulance to the hospital from where he never returned. She walks without an expression using a walker. She does not make eye contact with any one, nor does she say hello to anyone. She bears a grim disposition. It seems she dislikes being seen using a walker because walkers are supposed to be for very old people. She seems determined to get well, and in this pursuit she never misses her daily ritual of walking and making an effort to walk faster. But often she forgets the way to the elevator to her apartment, and then she is compelled to break her silence by asking someone about the elevator banks. I admire her because she is trying to cure herself, and in this vein she is trying her best.

After a few days of stroke, I could not recognize the English Language, and of course I could not understand most of the spoken words on TV, It was burdensome just to look at TV. Imagine, what other people must be thinking of me: Einstein? Later, driving was a definite challenge. Recognizing the Exit and taking it successfully became a difficult proposition. I used to see the exit but fail to recognize it, in time, to be the one for me to take. The message of right exit was either not reaching the brain, or not being processed fast enough to tell me yes go ahead and take it. Often, I had to try a few times, even if I was around my home. The visual message took a very long time to get registered and processed by the Brain which had lost Memory. The result was delay in executing the turn became a common happening.

To learn English language, once again, I started to watch news and my favorite old movies every day. I spent as much time as my energy and vision allowed me to. And then I started to spend considerable time on the internet as well. In the beginning, it was hard for me to focus longer than just a few minutes at a time, but gradually I succeeded in developing the habit of spending more time on TV and Internet. When loss of vision, memory, and comprehension are at very low levels, then concentration becomes difficult and tiredness is resulted. I chose the programs and web-sites that interested me, and that gave me the incentive to spend all the time I could. Constant viewing helped me to regain a lot of my memory, recognition of spoken words, English text, humor, vocabulary, etc., while there were other things that I just could not recall or learn for quite some time. Thanks to my Internet Service Provider who happens to be WebTV. WebTV provides internet service through the television. They provide a monitor to hook up with the TV and the viewer can use remote key pad as well remote monitor. The print and the page are quite large to view from a distance. I would recommend web TV to all patients, because it helped me to relearn a lot of things once again. Practice, practice, and patience, patience became my motto …

Amazingly, I had forgotten how to WALK, All these physical difficulties were not making me sad and pitiful, but on the contrary they were creat-ing a lot of HUMOR in my mind, and often I used to laugh at my follies, privately of course. When I had to hold the hand-rails of the 5 steps down from my apartment to the sidewalk, I used to burst out in laughter, think-ing how useless and stupid I had become. I remained that way for may years. I started comparing myself with the under-nourished, weak, and sickly pony whose limbs and joints were out of control, and moving with-out coordination. In fact, my knees, ankles, hip, and shoulders were all behaving in a very funny way, and several other people commented on it, and this very thing started me to walk for at least one hour every night (after 9 or 10 pm) when no one was there to notice my super fashionable walk.. I was wobbling and swaying in every sense of the word. I used to laugh at my self because I was walking so funny, and I am sure I was a source of amusement for others who happen to watch me. I walked every day. I started to walk faster in subsequent months, but was unable to walk straight, and somehow the direction of walk used to swerve either to the left or right involuntarily. Later, I wanted to run, but after taking the left foot up I did not know what to do next. It took me quite a long time before I learned to coordinate alternate leg movements without breaking the pattern. It can be a difficult exercise, but it has got be done and all stroke patients should work on trying continuously. Just don't give up. If it feels like a punishment then let it be a punishment. Punishments do produce some good results and those are the good things we are looking for, no matter how small they may be.

With each little improvement there was a sense of accomplishment in me. This encouraged me, and made me try the next steps. It was learning process and I continued it. Here is something that I tried on myself. If you have walking difficulties then take your left foot forward and keep it firm on the ground and don't move it. Now lift your right foot and move it forward and place it right in front of the left foot. At this moment both feet are on the ground. Stay in this position for a few seconds. Now lift your left foot once again and place it right in front of the right foot. Stay in this position for a few seconds. This walking exercise will seem like a walk in slow motion. Like a robot you repeat putting each foot forward right in front of the other, and maintaining that position for a few seconds and then repeating the routine once again. You will develop control, coordination, and balance at the same time. Do not speed up the exercise process even if you are sure that you can. Do this exercise several times, for a few days, and surprise yourself with your renewed walking capability,

ENERGY & STRENGTH were some of the key factors without which even my built up public image of being in good health were failing.

Instead of gaining strength and energy, I seemed to be losing them. Here are some of things I started to do. I took a light weight book in my left hand and twisted my hand in various ways then I did the same thing with my right hand for a couple of days. Later I graduated this little exercise to move my wrists and arms in as many ways as I could do. Surprisingly enough even a quarter pound book can feel heavy when you do not have strength in your body. I maintained this exercise routine with heavier books, and it felt better each week. After about 15 months, I went to buy dumbbells. I had great difficulty in lifting 15 lb. dumbbells from the store rack in to the shopping cart, and later to load them in my car. My mind was strong but the body was not. In subsequent months I tried different exercises which are commonly known. To develop energy, I had learned as a young athlete that a lot of liquids, vegetables, fruits, some grains, less sugar, some protein combined with activity will boast the energy levels. So I carried out this diet practice with a lot of pacing the carpets in my home and outside. Make your own choices of nutritious foods from the non animal food source and drink a lot of water with whatever activity you can get involved in so far it involves walking. Just make sure that you eat in small portions only. Soon you will find that your energy levels are much higher than before.

Another very important area that must be looked at by stroke and heart patients, and non patients and, that is, the **TOES** which are generally in the socks and shoes. We do not see our toes all the time, and we take it for granted that they are all right. Reduced circulation of blood in the body may not supply enough blood to the toes which will become pink and then red gradually. If not attended by a physician right away, this condition can mature to gangrene. Some physicians will only check the blood pressure at the top of the ankle and at the beginning of the toes, and if the pressure is acceptable then they would tend to ignore the pink or red toes. During several medical checks over the years, I had my red toes seen by the doctors, and they went through the normal routine of checking the blood pressure on the ankle and the beginning of my left toe which used to get numb during the winter time, but no diagnosis were made. In fact as I write this line, I still have the red/blue blemish on the tip of my left toe. It still becomes numb during winter, and also when I do not walk for a few days in a row. Studying your own body and its symptoms will be beneficial for you, and help you in dealing with your physician in an intelligent way. Specific questions about specific physical condition will compel the doctor to give out specific answer. If you do not receive the right answer to your question, or do not feel satisfied, then ask the question in another form once again, and then again, until you feel satisfied. At times, you may realize an important question or explanation upon returning home, then do not hesitate to call the doctor's office at the first available opportunity to get the answers. Repeat calling your doctor until you feel satisfied.

Patients and non patients who end up preparing themselves before visiting their doctors, and ask pertinent questions, send a clear signal to the doctor that they want to get better as soon as possible, and do not want to get in to the habit of repeating such visits endlessly. Before each visit, prepare a list of questions for which you want definite answers. In this way, you will not forget any thing to ask. You want to get well, and stop visiting the doctor thereafter, except for periodic check ups. You do not want to be the doctor's calendar filler. You have got your health condition under control, and then you want to stop visiting the doctor over and over again for the same ailment. I will provide reasons to justify the need for your active participation in your own well being, and the expeditious conclusion of visits to your doctor once the health condition gets under control. Various studies indicate that more than 150,000 Americans die, each year, from medical mistakes. This is a conservative number which, in fact, could reach up to 200,000 or more. Somehow, the general public is more concerned about high costs of medical services and drugs, along with the influence of insurance companies in the provision of medical services. Various reasons could be attributed to such a high number of medical error related deaths every year and they could be over work, lack of experience, lack of proper focus, shortage of trained nurses, over worked healthcare workers in general, insufficient time spent with the patient, carelessness, irresponsibility, etc.

Additionally, there is another danger being in the hospital or doctor's clinic which is catching infections and viruses from the environment of such facilities. When there is a shortage of trained nurses and other qualified healthcare staff, it is likely that patients and non patients to get injured within those facilities. Also, it is very easy to get infections from these medical facilities where all kinds of diseases are treated. It is an environment of infections. Patients and non patients do not need such headaches.

I experienced a very strange thing, and that was about my memory. A large amount of my memory related to recently learned names, experiences, techniques, skills, etc. was lost with varying degrees. I felt that way, because I could not recall them. In the beginning, I could not recognize the English language, besides reduced vision. Absolutely, I was unable to remember any names, towns, etc. The streets, locals, and scenes of immediate vicinity became somewhat strange looking to me. I remember after several months of stroke occurrence, I used to take a short drive, but returning used to become a challenge. I used to return home after making stops to rest and get my bearings in tact, but even then it was an ordeal to remember the streets and turns. Upon seeking help with driving directions to my home, I faced another challenge, and that was to remember the directions given, which I used to forget within a minute or just before reaching my car, and this condition lasted for at least 5 years. Just do not feel shy to ask for help whenever you happen to be lost, or need direction, or need any kind of help. Children do not feel shy; whenever, they want something they just ask, and whenever they are uncomfortable they just complain, so and so forth. Ask for help like children do. After all, after a stroke, mind and body are hardly functional, with almost no energy, similar to that of a child. To have a shower in the morning, which has been my daily ritual, I had to reconfigure the way to maneuver bathroom tub faucet and to set the correct water temperature for a very long time. And this was the scenario in almost everything I attempted to do even if it was a repeat experience. I had to reconfigure. Nature subjected me to go through that routine during and after my subsequent stroke experiences. For about 8 years during and after the strokes I bought several pairs of pants and only recently I realized that each one of them is at least 2 inch shorter. Until recently, I thought that they were of the right length (an example of stroke aftermath). Others looked at my pants and then looked at my face, but I never understood the thought behind their expressions. Each time I remember these moments, I acceptingly laugh at myself. We do end up doing a lot to survive each and every day of our short span of life. We should be thankful for each effort we are able to make on our own toward survival on daily basis.

One typical example that I can offer is that I could not retain the message of locking my front door before going out for a walk. After taking just a few steps out, I had to return to check if I had locked my door. Sometime, I used to return to my door to check the lock for about 10 times, mostly about 5 times. The same was the case with my car. Now, after 10 years of major stroke experiences, with mild ones in between, I have improved tremendously. I still return to my front door or car door at least once to check the locks. I have improved tremendously. I am thankful to the people who laughed at my foolish behavior and foolish conversation, whether in front of me or behind me, and I am thankful to myself because I enjoyed my follies too, because it reinforced the thought of healing myself just as fast as it was possible. Often, I laugh at my follies, sometime shamefully.

All these experiences taught me to look after myself and to survive. I learnt that during a desperate health condition, getting better is the only issue at hand, and it requires as much focus as your energy levels allow you to provide. Stroke occurrence is not a crime, and has never been one. Be open in describing your physical and mental health problems, depending upon your capability at a given time, and let people know about it. If people scoff, laugh, or ignore you then you know who not to ask for help. Meaningful help that a stroke or heart patient requires can only be given by people who understand the patients' problems and needs, and among these people the ones who have compassion and care giving intentions and capability are the only ones, including physicians, who count. Qualified and experienced doctors who happen to possess the deep seated compassion, caring, affection, pain, pity, and a great degree of compulsion to save and cure the patient are probably the most humane and appropriate doctors for the stroke and heart patients. They are rare. Acknowledgement of human dignity becomes acutely important when a doctor takes care of male and female patients of all ages, ethnicities, colors, faiths, economic levels, and provides them with the needed care and attention.

Unfortunately, in today's world, the cost of operating a medical service, with numerous legalities, is so high that the billing aspect of patient care becomes important and consequently healthcare providers end up making choices and preferences which happen to be completely contrary to the main issue of saving and curing stroke and heart patients. We live in competitive and commercial system. Almost everything is about making money. Medical practitioners are a part of this system, and they want to make money just like anyone else. Now, how to connect two very different needs. Medical practitioners are in business and provide healthcare as their service product; stroke and heart patients require immediate focused care where every minute or even a second becomes crucial for the well-being of the patient. Medical practitioners are bound if not compelled at times, to set priorities which may not be in the best interest of a patient. In some cases, at least, money may play a part; while in other cases gender, race, accent; color, looks, etc. may play a significant role. It is a riddle that is becoming more complex every year. How can anyone conceive that the Medical professionals do not require a decent life style; they need as much a good life as anyone else, may be a bit more, but not beyond more and beyond the need of patients well being.

The moment some professional is in business, then the survival of business becomes of prime importance, which is very legit as well as natural. When the highways are built and trucking companies start hauling freight, the railways get hurt and therefore do not like to see highways and the automobile industry to flourish. Because, this development is contrary and competitive to the interests of railways, it becomes obvious for them to dislike it. Who can blame the railways for harboring such a self protective intention? Similarly, pharmaceutical companies would not like if someone can come up with the idea of developing some herbal remedy which costs pennies as compared to expensive drugs produced by them. Pharmaceutical companies want to sell their products, and do not want competitive circumstances. **Brain surgery, heart surgery, triple bypass, organ transplants, etc. are all businesses for the surgeons,** and in no way they want to lose their business. Instead, surgeons promote their services through out the medical community in one way or another. The moment a stroke or heart patient arrives at a clinic or hospital, he or she becomes a potential client for a variety of services which are essentially formulated to help the patient, while at the same time the patient's arrival becomes a big signal for big dollar amount. The big dollar amount is deeply associated with the medical community.

We know that medical community is in business, and they got to make money to survive. In view of this fact, just visualize that why wouldn't they want to expand their business with any patient who arrives at the clinic with stroke or heart condition. Of course, the medical community does take full advantage of such an opportunity, because they are in business to help the patient. Possibly most people around the world have clogged arteries to some degree or so. The accepted guidelines provide the doctors to perform necessary surgery under certain circumstances. Suppose the patient falls under those guidelines which may warrant triple bypass surgery, then the doctor is obliged and free to perform the surgery or send the patient to the specialist who would perform the surgery. Doctor will save the patient's life, and for this purpose will send the patient to the specialist for the surgery. Patient has just to be within those guidelines. Therefore, it is strongly recommended that patients and non patients should be visiting doctors regularly, so that any diagnosis may be received in writing while the patient has complete comprehension capabilities. Just avoid being in unconscious state and being brought to the clinic for medical help. Stay pro-active regarding your health, and recognize the importance and value of being able to manage all your health related visits to your doctor by yourself. Try your best to be in conscious state when you visit your doctor or the hospital emergency ward, because you will not be able to make any decisions if you are unconscious.

Medical community is under pressure to produce profits, as well as, help the patient. This is a complicated process with extreme conflictions. Patient wants to survive and get better, and doctor wants to help but want to make money. Here the patient and non patient should exercise his or her involvement vigorously. No one should be able to take something out of your body, or implant in your body without your complete agreement and control. Percentage of good and bad doctors and percentage of honest and dishonest doctors is proportionate to the similar attributes in the specific population. If your town has 20% of dishonest people, then most likely you will end up having at least 20% of dishonest doctors. Equally, if your town has 15% percent of incompetent people, then it is likely that you will end up having at least 15% of the incompetent doctors. Business environment remains about the same in most businesses. Businesses do not like competition, do not want to lose business, and most definitely want to maximize their specific services to obtain more profits. The only resort a stroke or heart patient or a non patient has is to be aware of the medical condition, as well as, the doctor's approach to the issue. Do not hesitate to ask questions, and then question again. Normally healthy people and the patients should make a note that they should avoid parking their body in the medical workshop for any length of time. In fact, they should refrain from doing so, unless there is no way out due to the severity of medical condition.

From time to time just about all of us have received advice to find a 'good' lawyer, 'good' accountant, 'good; mechanic, 'good' doctor, etc, and we do end up having one and trust develops over a period of time, thereafter everything seems to move smoothly. Realistically, good doctors are not always available in the neighborhood. Therefore make your doctor a good doctor by taking charge of your health affairs. To overcome the probability of having a bad experience with your doctor, nurse, or the hospital of your choice, the most important thing that I can suggest is to become the manager of your body and health. Even though you may have a high regard for your doctor and treat him or her with extreme respect, which should be the case with all of us, make sure that you know exactly what is being said, what is exactly being done to your body, and what advice and medication you are receiving in such a process. Questions and answers should be exchanged for as long as you feel they are necessary. You cannot change the system, it is not feasible to find the ideal doctor who is located near your home, etc., and in view of this the best thing you can do is to accept the doctor you have and manage your treatment with your doctor's help.

The current health system has got to be reconfigured, so that money, which is an enormous amount, does not play a key role in the provision of healthcare, instead healthcare should be provided entirely for the reasons of well being of the total population. A good healthcare system is essential for the survival of a social system, and therefore should not be based entirely on commerce. Commerce based healthcare system will not only bring dissatisfaction but also chaos and disgruntlement. Such dissatisfied and antagonizing feelings can eventually hit home and can disrupt even a great civilized society. After all healthcare is as close an issue to all humans as anything can be. **Healthcare is not a commercial or a political issue; it is a human issue.** Adequate healthcare should be mandatory in any civilized society, and no one should be left uncovered. Virus from one person can reach all of the rest of the population, and we should not be able to use the excuse that, 'that' person was not treated because 'that' person did not have health insurance. One sick person without healthcare can unintentionally wipe out a good segment of the population. President's constitutional duty is to protect the people of the USA, and in the same vein it is his duty to protect all people through universal healthcare insurance.

We must realize that stroke or heart attack occurrence requires immediate medical attention. Stroke or heart attack is a condition which deteriorates the brain and body on a continuous basis and to some extent even after the medical attention has been provided. All of us should make it a point to treat our mind, body, and the soul with respect, and should make all the effort to safeguard them. We provide so much attention to our car or TV when it is being repaired, because we are very curious as to the outcome of such repairs, and if such repairs would provide the same quality of stimulus as before. We do not provide same level of care and attention to our body. We tend to abuse our body with no mercy, while we will do extremes to see that our cars are in good shape. If we are knowledgeable about the car, then it becomes easy to manage its maintenance, repairs, and able to effectively deal with the mechanic who is repairing it. Similarly, if we are knowledgeable about stroke and heart disease, then we can manage it and effectively deal with it ourselves and through the medical community.

Amazingly enough, while my immediate memory was almost lost, my memory of distant past became very acute and I could vividly remember the faces, conversations, names, incidents, jokes, etc., in complete details, which I had forgotten entirely over a period of time. The names and faces of my primary school classmates became vivid in my mind. All the vocabulary of other languages that I had learned as a young boy and as a young man became available to me clearly. I thought that I had completely forgotten these languages. Since, my contact with the public was quite limited, I spent much time in dreaming or watching TV. I was surprised to find myself solving mathematical problems almost instantaneously on the learning channel. I could reach the correct answer, but could not figure out the process, or path to such solutions. My surprise was primarily due to the documented fact that mathematics was not one of my favorite subjects.

MEMORY DEVELOPMENT

I developed my own memory exercises. Counting 1 to 100 was almost a height of excellence for me at that time, and even later. So I started out counting up to 20, and later I gradually increased it to 100. After 10 years,

I can't say if the difficulty is entirely over. Occasionally, I do have difficulty in going forward after counting up to 60. I used to pour 4 to 5 cups of fresh water in the coffee pot every morning; and often I had to throw out the water and count again. So I counted out loud, and eventually the problem went away. Now, whenever I experience a problem of keeping a visual thought for more than a minute, I speak it out.

Like after locking the front door, I used to return to the door again and again to make sure it was locked, so I started to write first and later started to speak out: "the door is locked". Here the problem is quite simple: retention of thought for at least 2 minutes. Once I learnt to keep the thought that the door was locked for just 2 minutes, I felt free to depart for my destination. Other exercises were to remember other people's names, telephone numbers, trying to remember different and new subjects, so on and so forth. Small steps like these work, and to accomplish these with favorable results, one does not need outside help. Patients' can experiment and get accustomed to these in a very short time. Just remember that you are trying to get better and you happen to be in charge, and the caregivers, doctors, loved ones happen to be just helping you to take charge and get better.

ANGER MANAGEMENT

Another significant aspect of stroke experience was that I found it to be extremely difficult to pull myself out of thoughts relating to Anger. I felt that the feeling of anger was like a trench and I happened to be in it where I happened to be trapped and was unable to pull myself out. After realizing that this feeling of anger will take me to a stroke occurrence, I used to try to shake it off somehow. This was not an easy task for me. Anger is like a deep trench and the patient gets stuck in it from where it is very difficult to climb out. In order to shake the feeling of anger, I used to get out of bed, pull myself of deep sleep, leave the house, throw cold water on my face continuously, shout, sing, rub the side of sofa, eat chips, etc. It took a lot of work, but I have learned it and now I can shake off my anger almost all the time successfully. Additionally, I started to learn to avoid having hostile thoughts, and instead of delving in to anger I started to concentrate on the root causes of anger. I learned to postpone the responses to any aggravating circumstances, and adopted a 'sit on it' position for a few days. I learned to be tolerant and forgiving, non combative, and bit more peaceful than I was before. Anger is basically unproductive and in fact does not say anything to meet your demands at that moment. If we end up forming specific questions and demands that would satisfy our needs, as long as they are within reason, then the anger could be transformed in to a quest. Ask questions and demand the unfulfilled commitments. This will take you to the next phase which will require decision making. At that time, you will either go forward with the choice of decision or retreat from the issue. At least, you have taken a step forward from the state of anger. In most cases, the moment you reach the position that is created by your questioning and your demands, your anger will be diffused. You will feel that you are out of that trench. Now you will be at a new position "should I call the police", or "ask a friend for help", or "file a law suit', or "write to some higher authority', or something like that. Alternatively, you may decide that any of those choices may not be worth the money and the effort and consequently forget the whole thing. So in this case, you moved from anger to decision making stage and by doing so you have potentially averted a possibility of stroke or a heart attack.

SELF HYPNOSIS

The most successful counter thoughts that worked for me were: Why do I need to burn myself out before the actual time? Why should I hurt myself for nothing by thinking these thoughts? I am punishing myself for money. I do not need that money which my business partner is stealing from me, this could be a signal for me to change the line of business or, what goes around does come around and everybody will be paid according to their deeds, I will get well, I am working on getting well each day, I am gaining strength, I can read, I can make my own breakfast, so and so forth. This may work for you or may not. Do make an attempt to make something like this to suit your particular situation, and speak the chosen words out loudly several times (in your home). You will be surprised to experience the positive results. This is a kind of self hypnosis. Self hypnosis works, and you can customize and develop your own.

Sometimes, we have to extend these hypnotic sermons to others. Lester, my neighbor at that time had a stroke and after hospitalization, he returned with a tube in his nostrils and a walker, and his speech was just a slur, his left side from head to his leg was affected. After knowing him for 6 months in this condition, I started to tell him that he did not look good using a walker. I repeated this for several weeks, and then one day he shouted a hello at me with a stick waving to me. He had left the walker behind. He was happy. About six weeks later, I started to ridicule him for using the stick when he could walk without it, of course in a jovial manner. One day, I asked him to show me the stick, and he handed me his stick which I placed at about 15 yards away, and asked him sternly to come and get it. In just 3 to 4 tries, he was walking without the stick, and each time he saw me he laughingly yelled at me "I do not use a walking stick any more". He pushed himself, learned it how to get out of it, and freed himself of continuous dependence. I felt real good, and that is what we all seek: "feeling good".

Without proper pronunciation, it will be difficult if not impossible to comprehend what the patient is saying. If others are unable to understand what the patient is saying, then the well wishers can only guess. If the guess is right then all goes well, however, if the guess is wrong and the patient is misunderstood, this state of communication can make the patient irritable and helpless. Irritability and helplessness are very bad for the patient's recuperation efforts, and a super stress could get accumulated to cause another stroke or heart attack. Instead of totally depending upon other people for every thing or any thing, I strongly suggest that patients should be practicing relearning vocabulary and the pronunciation of the words just as soon as it is possible. Speech, pronunciation, and later writing are the communication tools to interact with other people and, therefore, they are absolute essential elements of our existence in an organized society.

Even if other people are involved in the process of relearning speech, pronunciation, and writing, the ultimate impact and responsibility of the borrowed learning falls on the patient. So, why not be proactive, and start doing something right away or as soon as it is physically and mentally possible. Delays in implementing such self exercises would only deteriorate the ill effects of stroke or heart attack. Be determined to do it yourself, and do not wait for someone to write a prescription for learning help for another day. Here are a couple of suggestions from my own personal experience. To shake off **STRESS** from your life is easier said than done. However, there is an ancient breathing remedy which may provide some relief from stress at least for a short period of time. Take a deep breath from your nose or mouth; hold it for a few moments then release it through the nostrils quickly with a moaning sound. Repeat this exercise several times, and each time make a moaning sound as you exhale through the nostrils. This exercise does work and it can be carried out as often as it is comfortable for you to do so for some positive outcome. After a couple of times, you will feel some relief from the stress. There are several breathing exercises that can help patients, and they require learning from a teacher. There are several Yogic exercises on breathing, which have proven to be beneficial for thousands of years. Walking, light exercise, meditation, social interaction, etc. are some of additional stress relieving methods.

To improve speech, first make these sounds: Ooooooooooo, Aaaaaaaaaaa, Eeeeeeeeeee, Awaaaaaaaa,, Heeeeeee,, and Hhaaaaaaaa in as loud a manner as you possibly can. To avoid commotion, carry out these exercises in the privacy of your room or the bathroom, but do let people know in some way that this is going be exercise, and not a call for help. Secondly, open your mouth and insert a portion of your fist and keep it under a biting position underneath your teeth. This will compel the mouth to stay open. If you find any discomfort, then bring portion of the fist out, but let it remain in the same position, thereby lowering the size of the bite. In this position, you will not be able to speak. The only thing you will be able to do is to produce a hoarse sound. Keep the fist in the mouth and make as loud a noise as you can. Repeat it as many times as you feel comfortable with. Graduate to the third stage quickly, which is to keep the portion of the fist in your mouth and say A, B, C, D, E, so on and so forth. In fact, doing this everyday will do you a load of good in your speech improvement. From this exercise, you can go to the next one at your own speed, and at your own leisure. The next exercise is to keep the portion of the fist in your mouth, and say 1, 2, 3, 4, 5, 6, so on and so forth. I know that these exercises are easy to recommend but difficult to carry out. Whether you succeed in performing these exercises correctly or not, but trying them every day will do you good. You will find the improvement in your speech inside a few weeks time. To achieve these results you do not require anyone but your own self.

Relearning pronunciation of words require practice too. The practice to relearn the pronunciation requires hearing the words in correct pronunciation. You may want to have your hearing checked out by a speech and hearing clinic. As we grow old we do experience some hearing loss. Under normal conditions, this hearing loss is only in very low frequency regions of sound. When we are very young, all the frequencies of sound can be heard. But we grow old, and some of it is lost. So, it will be a good idea to have your hearing checked. If there are some recommendations and prescriptions from the speech and hearing clinic, then do follow them. For a new patient fresh from a stroke or heart attack experience, any and every noise is annoying. They want quiet all around them. After a little while, the patients seem to accept conversational sounds coming from people around them, or even a T.V. After the patient gets accustomed to the sounds without getting annoyed by them, it is a perfect time to gradually bring conversation in to the patient's life. We must remember that hearing, speaking, and writing require memory, and its connection to the ears, vocal chords, mouth, eyes, hands, fingers, etc. which got damaged during the stroke or heart attack occurrence. We are trying to rehabilitate a damaged condition to a workable condition. This process requires patience, determination, and continuous enthusiasm to be able to prove fruitful.

In my case, I started with TV, but the noise surrounding the vocal and pictorial parts of what was on the screen became overbearing. First of all I could not see the images on the screen clearly. Most of time, I could only see the forms of people on the screen, and not the complete face with its features. Most of what was said used to pass by me like a breeze. I could understand some of the spoken words, but just for a few moments, and then reach a blank state. This I learned later to be because I could not retain anything that I heard and, therefore, could not process it. Whatever I did understand was just for a moment only, and also I could never remember that after just a little while. Also, change of scene on the TV screen, every few seconds was too much for me to handle. Due to the noise, not understanding what was being said, not being able to see clearly, and a host of other problems made me to shut the TV off and without fail it brought peace to my little world.

The need to develop vision, relearn English speech, understanding, spelling, vocabulary, writing, etc. diverted me to the Internet. Internet became a real tool for me to learn a lot of things without too much noise, changing screens, etc. I relearned a lot from the Internet, and I continue to do so. Of course, my verbal and written exchanges with the people were another story, an embarrassing one to say the least, but I have crossed it somehow. You will too, if you keep at it.

While reading, whether it is on the internet or a written material, repetitive reading of the same paragraph is recommended to start with. Each time you read, you might understand it somewhat differently. Try to remember this repeatedly read written material after a few minutes, after an hour, after several hours, and the next day. The written material being read should be of prime interest of the patient. These interests could be fashion, dress style, jewelry, cartoons, jokes, romance, crime, science, religion, politics, travel, sports scores, etc. Now, try to read as much as it is comfortable to do so, every day, and confirm to your self as to what and how much you retain of what you read. If your retention of reading material happens to fall in specific area, then it is the most appropriate area to read more than other areas. Make sure that you discipline yourself to set a time to recollect what you had read a few hours before or a day before. Another exercise in this area of short term memory development as well as relearning the reading abilities is to try to read about a specific topic presented by different internet websites or different writers. Just like various newspapers have different views about the same subject matter, you will be able to see several such possibilities in respect to any subject on the internet. These exercise methods will speed up your comprehension, relearning of English language, spellings, and short term memory. By the way, I still have problems with the spelling of words and grammar. There are days when I have almost none, and yet there are days when I have more than I ever expect them to be.

After a short while, start reading loudly, even just for a few minutes. If the words do not come out freely, then push the words out somehow, even if you have to exert a bit. The most important thing here is the formation of words which, at first, will be slow and then timely. Once the words are formed in your mind to use for a certain piece of conversation, you have already accomplished the most important task. Now to take it out properly is to complete the process. Try forcing these words out, no matter what you have to do, and what embarrassing moments you have to experience. Before long you will be doing this just normally, and gaining on relearning of your normal speech capability. Forming of specific words is important because without these words, we end up waiting, searching in our mind, and possibly stuttering. If possible, try to get hearing and speech therapy from a medical university nearby you. I took it, and it helped me.

Unless we hear correctly, it will be difficult to reproduce vocally in a correct manner, if not impossible to do so. Speech is directly related to hearing. If the hearing is good then the speech is good, and visa versa. You already know that when English language is taught by a native English speaker from England, the pupils will learn the English phonetics as they happen to be practiced in England. On the other hand, if the pupils are being taught English by American teacher then they will speak in American phonetics. Now if during the process of relearning of English language, and you happen to have a caregiver who has minimal educational level and poor command of English language at best, then the exercise of making conversation with that person may end up producing negative results for you. You being a stroke or heart attack recovering patient with speech and memory disability, then even listening to the caregiver's inadequate and broken English will prove to be negative. I would call it a disservice to patients. This listening of inadequate and broken English could make the patient annoyed, irritated, and lead the patient to feel aggravated and helpless. I have witnessed such scenes at numerous times, and I see them now. The healthcare provided caregivers do not seem to have much sympathy for the patient who is like a vegetable sitting in a wheelchair, waiting for the day to be over, while the caregiver is busy talking to her family or friends on the cell phone providing all kinds of wrong English words, pronunciations, grammar, and noise to the patient's ears.

Here is a scenario that you, your loved ones, well wishers, and healthcare providers should not let the patient get exposed to. Patient cannot speak properly, or is extremely weak, does not know how to exercise his or her choices and preferences, feels grateful that one human body is there to lift him or her in case of fall, etc. Instead of receiving developmental help, the patient ends up receiving a health worsening support. If you happen to be in such a situation, then do think about it, and go through various steps to raise this issue to every one, no matter how disconnected they might be. Just start voicing your choices and preferences to whosoever comes near you. If the doctor or nurse comes near you, before any other conversation or procedure, raise your issues. Just say that you are not comfortable with whatever things you are not comfortable with.

Talking about Self Hypnosis, during these several years of getting better I read several books on this subject some of which I had been taught as a young boy. As a young boy, I was taught that if anger resides in your brain then you do not need an outside enemy, which means that anger is the biggest enemy that humans can have. Somehow, we all harbor anger to some degree. I do not know if one can easily control it completely, but most definitely it is possible to reduce its intensity to a very low level where it is almost harmless. You can do it yourself in the privacy of your bed-room or wherever it is quiet and no one to disturb you for just 5 minutes. Sit in a comfortable position and close your eyes. Take several deep breaths and try to concentrate on your breathing only. Do not think anything else. Just focus on your breathing. You will feel at peace, or somewhat at peace. Divert your attention from your breathing to your mind and possibly to your forehead. Maintain the breathing rhythm. Start counting backwards from 30 to 1 (30, 29, 28, 27, 26.... to 1). Count in your mind and verbal-ize it also. Each time you count, just look at the number you are counting in your mind. When you say 30 look at the number 30 in your mind, when you say 29 look at 29 in your mind, when you say 28 look at the number 28 in your mind, ... and finally when you say 1 look at number 1 in your mind.

You should see 29 slightly at a lower level from 30, 28 is slightly at a lower level from 29, 27 is at a lower level from 28 .... and 1 is at lower level than 2. You are counting from 30 to 1 and continuously looking at the lower number as you say it out. You will be bringing your focus from 30 to 1 in a downward manner. You can start this exercise from 100 and downward, if you wish. Whatever number you feel comfortable with, just start from there. Exercise this for a couple of days, and see you are able to see the numbers in your mind as you speak them out. If you wish to speak out these numbers louder, it is even better. Just suit yourself.

After a couple of days exercise, just like before sit down and breath com-fortably for a minute or two and focus on your breathing only. Start counting downwards from 30 to 1 and looking at the specific number when you count that number. You may experience a feeling that your attention is traveling downward also. You will feel that your attention has reached from the higher level of your forehead to the point where your forehead meets the nose bone. After a few months, you could feel that this focus point will be even deeper than in the beginning sessions. Once you reach to 1 in your counting, visualize that there is big door in front of you. You open this door and go through it and reach a well decorated hallway with thick carpet. There is an elegant looking stairway. You take the stairway down and a group of people waiting to greet you. Most of them are known to you and some of them you are unable to remember. Among these people you will find the ones who hurt you, cheated you, hated you, etc., and gave you a lot of grief and anger. But here they are smiling at you in a loving manner and greet you with warmth you had not expected. You tell them that you do not hate them, and you are no longer angry with them, you forgive them all the way. Hearing these words coming from you, all of them feel relieved and each one of them hugs you and says goodbye in a loving way. You depart from them in a happy and peaceful way and go up the stairway, and open the door and go out. You are no longer angry. You can practice this exercise by focusing on individual basis. You can choose to visualize meeting just one person at a time, who had hurt you and had given you grief which resulted in anger. Forgiving this person and receiving that persons' acknowledgement will set you free of anger, possibly for ever. Forgive others before they get the chance to apologize to you. Such exercises will relieve you of the unnecessary expenditure of your mental energy which happens to be in a very short supply during the recovery period of stroke or heart attack experience.

Try doing this exercise every day, and you will come out of any anger. In similar way, you will be able to do so many good things that you choose to do for yourself. There are several other exercises which are a bit more complex than this one, and for which a complete recovery is required. Before, we can really cure the effects of stroke or heart attack, we must address a few issues, and resolve them to as much an acceptable degree as possible.

We all grieve a lot, even if something small happens that is contrary to the well being of our body. After the stroke or heart attack, most of us end up feeling why did it have to happen to me. I was in such a good shape, my whole life is affected, I am unable to do even the normal things, I am unable to work, I am out of money, I will not be able to support my family, I do not have enough money to get well, I do not have enough insurance to pay for the medication, I do not have medical insurance, etc.

Some form of anger sets in. It does not seem fair, I cannot perform, I cannot think, I cannot remember, I cannot speak, I cannot walk, loved ones and others think I have gone loco, no one wants to be near me, I have become a burden on others, etc. Anger and irritability become every day challenge for the patients. They are part of our personalities and we cannot shake them off easily. But we can subdue and make them a lesser burden and nuisance, and more importantly a lesser danger to our health. Out of control anger can be life threatening for stroke and heart patients. Stroke and Heart patients have limited capabilities to control anger. Therefore, the caregivers, loved ones, and the doctor must make deliberate effort to see that stroke patients do not get aggravated or irritated for any reason for quite some time, at least until the patients somewhat recover from the first difficult phase of stroke or heart attack occurrence. Besides learning to control the irritability and anger on daily basis through self control, self hypnosis, philosophizing, meditation, etc., patients can practice a very easy method of releasing anger. While in privacy of bedroom or bathroom, patients may let out a single note utterance in somewhat loud manner. In other words, patients may loudly say: "Aaaaaa ………", or "Ouuuuuuuuuuu ………", or "Godddddddd ………", etc. Just 15 to 30 seconds of this vocal outlet will make the patient comfortable. This method is a good way to release pent up energy produced by anger in our brain.

The most prominent irony and predicament of the circumstances faced by patients is that 1) stroke patients' brain and the inside of the body is reduced to somewhat that of a child, 2) doctors, loved ones, caregivers, and general public perceive him/her as an adult who thinks and performs as an adult, 3) stroke patient, himself or herself, thinks of himself and herself as adult who is capable of handling anything and everything as before. Once the patient realizes, through self realization only, that there are activities the patient can handle by him/her self, and to perform other specific activities he/she would require outside help. Once these two factors are determined in patients' mind, it becomes the beginning of taking control of getting well by the patient. Patients have got to control the process of getting well and once the boundary lines are identified in terms of what can be done without help, and what cannot be done without help, the focal point of development area becomes clear in patients' mind. It has been said that once we know our weaknesses, we come to know what needs to improve. Then the improving methods can be targeted and employed.

No work, no money, no friends, no conversations, no normal life, it will take a very long time to heal if at all, pitiable condition, helplessness ... thoughts like these will occupy the mind most of the time. Probably, these are the only thoughts damaged brain can present at that time; brain is attending to the immediate problems which are the effects of stroke or heart attack. Brain will continuously send signals for focus on damage and repair, which are the functions of brain.

DEPRESSION sets in. Depression is considered to be a major health problem today. It can trigger another stroke or heart attack, cause other diseases, and also can cause one to commit suicide, and so on. Depression must be handled immediately, with or without medication. Healing without medication will require a lot of self discipline, patience, self hypnosis, meditation, and good faith. But in the end you will come out completely healed, and in the process you will learn each step of such healing. This will enable you to go to that particular issue directly which requires re-visiting, should such a need arise in the future.

Some of the common symptoms of depression are: difficulty in sleeping at night, continuous sadness, lack of interest in any activity, feelings of failure, not interested in people and conversations, feelings of being trapped with no way out, feeling of life being unfair to you, feelings of constant fatigue, helplessness, waiting for life cycle to complete, feeling of being isolated, feeling of "nobody wants me", feeling of being useless and inadequate, lack of self confidence, avoiding people, and distrusting people at large.

Stroke or heart attack occurrence does damage the brain and the body. I would compare this damage to your being sent to 3rd grade from your current position of post graduate professor. The body and the emotions, and therefore the needs, become that of a young child. At least, it happened to me, and I studied my experiences in details. I felt like a child who was helpless and when I could not fulfill my needs right away I used to cry often, and sometimes for hours. To avoid the continual crying occurrence I started to watch cartoons, comedy, and animal shows on TV, and this diversion did help me tremendously. Not only I stopped daily crying regularly, but I started to take my condition humorously. This attitude lightened me up and, I think, it played a major role in my recuperation from the effects of stroke. Although I doubt very much if any body completely recovers from a few strokes or heart attacks ever, but getting better surely means that the patient is capable of essential functions of daily life, and is qualified to live the life that is available to the patient.

Besides, the body and mind are reduced to that of a child, hope, dreams, fantasies, and wishes just disappear, Fear of aging sets in. Loss of independence and lack of privacy become a daily issue. Self identity starts to decay due to lack of interaction, lack of normal daily functions, lack of routines, people walking away from you by using superficial one liners, etc. Your face and the expression become different. Your face is no longer the same face you used to be familiar with. Your facial expressions expel painful messages. Self esteem and self respect are extremely important part of our personality, and they play a very important role in every thing we do and achieve in our lives. After the stroke or heart attack, self respect and self esteem take a steep drop. All these aspects become crucial ingredients of Depression which is a killer in itself. First control Depression, and then cure it.

After stroke or heart attack occurrence, experiencing depression is almost a given thing. Do seek medical help, but do not give up trying to recognize it, control it, and cure it by yourself. After all in curing yourself of any physical or mental ailment, you are the chief participant and recipient of medical help, advice, therapy, and attention., and therefore your involvement and focus are crucial to your getting better and eventually cured. Do not hesitate to take control of the process of your getting better.

DEPRESSION can be recognized by you just by studying your own self for a number of weeks. After stroke or heart attack, patients do cry, feel helpless, feel friendless, experience disappearance of hopes and dreams, loss of independence, loss of privacy, fear of ageing, thoughts of death, thinking and thinking but of no substance or consequence, changes in facial features, weakness, disability, dependence, loss of self esteem, loss of self respect, lack of will, ego depletion, excessive crying, inability to concentrate, indifference to social activities and people in the environment, too little sleep, too much of eyes closed position but not sleeping, too much or too little appetite, unattended complaints of physical pains and uneasiness, too much anxiety and worrying about the least important things, feeling of being useless to every one around, too much irritability and experiencing anger at the slightest disagreement, experiencing thoughts of suicide and death.

Experience of depression after the stroke or heart attack is related to the same chemical imbalance causes depression in people who are not stroke or heart patients. This chemical imbalance which causes depression can affect our ability to think, reason, solve problems, and deal with people. So, depression can appear under both conditions.

Besides following the medical advice, do something for yourself in a complete voluntary manner. Try to devise your own strategy to get out of depression. Make it a project of your own, and start working on it. We are thankful when medical help, friends, loved ones, neighbors, and well wishers help us, but we should not wait for and depend upon their help alone;

we should do something ourselves by starting the process of getting well. Start filling up your calendar with activities, exercise walking, meeting people, going to parties and movies, reading, and participating in games. Try to develop programs and activities that stimulate you, and you look forward to their time and date to arrive. Additionally, develop activities for which you have to dress appropriately, For example, for walking, dancing, billiards, cards, dinner party, friends, romantic date, family, etc. one needs to wear appropriate clothes. Grooming and dressing up are positive steps toward getting out of any kind of depression.

Also, depression is closely related to continuously involved in thinking, whatever it may be. Just like feeling of anger in a patient's mind, or in the mind of a non-patient, the individual seems to fall in a trench of anger, and finds it difficult to get out of it, quite similarly thinking continuously for long periods of time become a difficult proposition to overcome. May be, it is a precursor to depression.

Feelings of **SEX** do not get disappeared after the stroke or heart attack, but the functional capability is most definitely reduced. So spouses and lovers should make note of this, and should try to accommodate the Stroke patient. This is very important, because sexual rejection by the lover or the spouse can easily enhance the depth of depression the Stroke patient is suffering from. Sex must be talked and this may elevate the confidence level in the patient. Fear, anxiety, and possible embarrassment can become the source of lack of sexual activity. Openness, encouragement, cooperation, accommodation, and communication will tend to produce very positive results. Physical disability and Emotional disability go hand in hand after the Stroke. Various weaknesses generated by depression, stress, anxiety, lack of activity, etc. become much greater weaknesses after the Stroke occurrence. Sexual dysfunction is common after the Stroke due to physical damage as well as emotional one. Stroke is a big trauma, and it remains in our minds for a very long time, even during intimacy, foreplay or sexual act.

Here, I am going to suggest something that may be controversial for the liberal minded people, but I feel very strongly about it. Develop deep loving relationship with the opposite sex before attempting any sexual activity. Love is supreme, and if you love her or him then you will be able to overcome any inadequacy in a variety of spheres that encompass relationship between man and a woman. Also, we must remember that love provides self respect, pride, responsibility, caring, self esteem, etc., beside the stimulation of hormones in the body. On the other hand, sexual activity with people who do not mean much creates reciprocal circumstance. They do not care for you either. Where does it land you? For a very short time, the ego may get a brief boost, but in the long run, it becomes a component of self disrespect which gets accumulated over a period of time and produces a basketful of psychological problems. Also, once realization hits you that you are not the most preferred partner, it may give you a sense of rejection which you do not need at this time. These accumulated psychological problems become a key factor in broken relationships, dissatisfaction with life, aimlessness, sadness, depression, etc. in the future and becomes a permanent feature of personality.

One way to outgrow from sexual dysfunctional state is to discuss everything with the spouse or lover. Once you are open, discussions do take place, thoughts get exchanged. Hidden fears tend to become components of such conversational thoughts, and consequently the details surrounding sex are exchanged, resulting in ventilation of sexual fears. Emotional problems can lead to impotency due to personality change, and depression. Poor self image is a significant factor in losing interest in sex. Bladder or bowl problem, common among Stroke patients, can produce awkwardness during sex, which reduces self image and, in turn, reduces interest in sex. Besides, many medications have side affects which do reduce libido. Remember that Stroke does not mean that you cannot have sex. Have it any way, whether your performance is good or not. Just do it and the evaluation portion of the equation can come some other day. Free your mind, and approach the one you really love. Love can overcome sexual dysfunction. We should never forget one thing and, that is, sex without love is a complete waste, and in my opinion should not be attempted, because doing so may lower your self esteem, lead to self criticism, and reduced sexual desire. Love is supreme, and sex is just a small portion of it. A complete and true feeling of love will provide the patients boundless ecstasy, and then it can be followed by sex. A complete and true feeling of love not only stimulates production of hormones, but it also relaxes the brain and the rest of the body. Mind feels secure and cared for. All body functions become normal with feelings of love which in most cases provides a glow on people's faces.

Talking to your spouse, lover, or the doctor could help solve the problem. Once the sexual fears are ventilated through open discussions, the patient is on the way to recovery from sexual dysfunction. It is a super therapy; it is self induced, private, inexpensive, and workable. Depression and lack of libido are very much curable with determined effort, will, participation and some spirituality. Yet, there are other alternatives to having sexual relationship with your significant other at a matured age. You may decide to learn the art and science of sublimation whereby you can divert the energy of instinct of sex to some other endeavors, causes, hobbies, etc. Millions of people have accomplished this sublimation through out the history. Additionally, consider the fact that nature provides sex for reproduction purposes only, and once that phase is over, then its importance is also minimized if not diminished entirely. All these and related thoughts may lead you to free yourself from the rituals, responsibilities, trials, emotional highs and lows, anxiety, etc. associated with it. Also, remember that you don't have to do any thing if you do not want to.

Anxiety is another significant factor that must be dealt with in a definite manner. From time to time, I wake up in the middle of night thinking that I am close to having another stroke or angina attack, and this creates a fear which prohibits me to go back to sleep. I become fearful that if something like this occurred during my sleep I would not be able to do anything for myself, so I remain awake. It could be the cause of tiredness, impatience, stress, etc.

The phenomena of emotional ups and downs should not be ignored, primarily due to the fact that it is a given condition after stroke or heart attack. From one level of emotion to another, like from laughter to anger suddenly, a sudden feeling of not being understood, or snubbed, or insulted, etc. In other words, mood swings take place on daily basis. Nutritious foods, rest, light and friendly conversation can stabilize the state of emotional ups and downs. In such light and friendly conversations, Stroke or heart patient should not be asked many questions, or none if possible. To respond to a question, the patient has to find an answer for which memory function will be required. Stroke damages the memory area of our brains. Patients find it difficult to retrieve vital data to answer the question, as part of this data has disappeared and other is very difficult to access. This can make the patient very irritable, and this irritation remains in the mind of the patient for a long time. It is possible that such irritations, if accumulated, can cause another stroke or heart attack without much delay.

We, as humans, are strictly social, and do everything with people. People are part and parcel of our lives. After stroke or heart attack, patients suffer from unpredictable behavior. Patients are unable to control their emotions, and on spur of the moment anger, hostility, tears, laughter, etc. can get triggered, and it can adversely affect the patients' chances of surviving in social and business world. Everything is connected with people, and the patients' world is adversely affected. Patient is isolated. In reality, the same people who depend on each other in every day life do not care, and do not tolerate if the patient is damaged, unable to operate, think, earn a livelihood, attract attention or love from the loved ones or anyone, for that matter. Consequently, patient's life becomes completely subjective and inverted, and it has got to be managed by the medical help, patient's own efforts, loved ones, and friends.

To cure this condition, step by step effort should be made to reduce, if not to eliminate, the factors that cause anxiety, stress, irritation, noise, questioning, depression, alcohol abuse, lack of self respect, etc. Outside help is always welcomed, however, self help and determination are key to getting well.

Often, care givers are assigned to patients who suffered severe physical and emotional damages after experiencing Stroke. And often, I have witnessed that care giver happens to be the least suitable person who should be near a stroke patient. Occasionally, after seeing a care giver accompanying a patient, I think the care giver needs a care giver. The care giver's minimum qualifications should be that he/she should be in good health, able to speak English or the language of the patient, should be of appropriate weight, and should be courteous, congenial, kind, caring, and sympathetic. Care giver should be able to understand patient's likes and dislikes, strong and weak points, and most definitely should be able to compliment the patient immediately upon the first available opportunity. Patient should be encouraged to perform various tasks where the patient has shown initiative or willingness. Compliments do make people happy, and the patients happen to be in desperate need of them. Besides compliments for very small accomplishments and tasks stroke the ego, and reinforces confidence to perform better. I like the idea of complimenting because this method is used in every kind of training process. Gently demonstrate the solutions of the patient's mistakes, and compliment patient's smallest acts. By receiving compliments, patients surmise that they are getting better, and the act of getting better motivates them to get to the next level of well being.

Patients should feel interested in getting better, and should manage the process of getting better. Do not hesitate to self monitor, self motivate, self evaluate, etc. at every level. After all it is your body, and it is your brain that needs to be healthy, and there is every reason to monitor and supervise it from one level to a higher level of betterment. For reading and spelling exercises, patients' will be better off choosing either audio or video separately. Newsprint is too small and therefore reading will be full of strain to the eyes and the brain. TV could prove to be alright provided reading on the screen and hearing somebody talk are not carried out at the same time. If the written material on TV or the Internet screen is being read by the patient, then the audio part should be minimized to silent, or to the minimum. Strangely, the audio can create difficulties in reading for the stroke patients, because they have limited energy, poor vision, and temporarily lost comprehension. Their attention will get too busy to perform the task of reading. We have recognized that one task and one accomplishment in the beginning is an adequate way to regain reading capability. Reading, listening, writing, spellings, etc. can be accomplished slowly, one issue at a time basis, successfully without overloading the patients' mind. Overloading patients' brain will fail, and it would result in patients to become irritated and angry which is a no, no. Writing will be another challenge. Finger tips may not be able to hold the pen in the right position for more than a couple of seconds, and the pen could slip. The hand and the arm will not go in the direction patients are writing, because muscle memory is lost. It will be difficult to recognize and read the hand-written script. Just take small steps to rectify this problem, and maintain positive attitude to overcome the difficulties. Several mini-steps like: writing one line at a time, and then stopping it. After a few minutes, write the second line, and stopping thereafter, so on and so forth. In this manner, the patients will be able to control the formation, legibility, and direction of writing straight on the line. This method is a significant source of encouragement for patients who see small accomplishments on regular basis, and will be tempted to write again to reach subsequent higher levels of accomplishments. For all these activities, patients do not require outside help; they can carry out these exercises on their own, at their convenience, and without extra noise and unwanted conversations.

We never realize how important each part of our body is until we nick ourselves with small cut on a finger or tow, or anywhere on the body. Normally, we are not aware that our whole body participates in the every activity of a day. When we experience a small cut on our finger, or anywhere on the body, somehow that portion of the body comes in to play so often each day that we are reminded of that cut through the pain and the lack of proper use of that limb. We seem unable to function properly just with a little cut. Now when the stroke occurs, the whole body and every function of it are adversely affected, while some functions are completely shut down. A cut on the finger is visible, but the damage as a result of stroke or heart attack is not visible (unless the blood is oozing out of head). The only visible part of stroke or heart attack is its affects. To view the location and specific damage, the patient has got to be scanned with sophisticated MRI, or similar, techniques.

One major challenge is faced by the stroke patient is **BALANCE**, which is essential for standing and numerous other activities. Once standing balance is intact then comes the walking part. Stroke patients are provided wheelchairs, and then walkers, or whatever the case may be, most suitable for the patient. I suggest that the patient should be brought alongside a solid steel railing and helped to stand next to it so that patient's weight is supported by the railing. Caregiver should keep the patient in that position, in comfort only, for a few minutes. Gradually, the patient should hold the railing, and after a series of similar exercises, on daily basis, the patient will develop a confidence to stand on his own by holding the railing as a support. Here the patient's desire, determination, and will to take control of his well being play a critical role. The next phase is when the patient is able to stand on his own without the support of the railing. Patient's subsequent stages will be progressively becoming independent of wheelchair and walkers, and graduating to walking stick which can be left behind also in a similar process of systematic exercises. Once the physical balance is regained, other areas of body functions get activated and become operational. Slowly but surely, the patient becomes independent.

For those patients who can stand and walk on their own, or have learned all these steps, the balancing exercise should be taken to the next level. Stand alongside the railing or a solid wall, hold the railing or wall with only one hand, left or right depending which side of the railing you are standing. Lift one leg and while holding the railing with one hand, keep standing on only one leg for a few minutes, or whatever time is comfortable for you. Repeat this exercise with the other leg. Switch the hands by getting on the other side of the railing or just turning yourself and facing on the opposite direction. The patient will become comfortable standing on one leg while using only one hand to hold the railing or wall, after a few exercises. Exercises must promote use of each leg separately. The next exercise is standing on one leg without holding the railing or wall. If the patient reaches one minute of free standing on one leg at a time, then he or she has accomplished something great. It is just one example of taking control of your getting better.

Simultaneously, you can add other exercises to restore BALANCE in other parts of the body. For example, you can fill a dish or a cup of water close to the brim of the dish or cup, and carry it across the room without spilling it. This will help increase the balance in walking, holding, and the direction of the walk. Additionally, this exercise will increase the mental focus and concentration which happens to be in desperately short supply after the occurrence of a stroke or heart attack. This is a helpful single physical activity which promotes balance, focus, and concentration at the same time.

One can progress to the next stage of walking exercise. Every one is familiar with the military soldiers marching in formation. Sometimes, these soldiers march very slowly, especially when they are marching for ceremonial reasons to honor some dignitary. They march very slowly. Each leg is put forward in a stiff manner very slowly, one after the other, while saluting toward the dignitary. It requires training beyond marching. It requires balance, control of leg muscles, feet, and perfect timing to perform the task of slow marching. Visualize this scene in your mind, and make an attempt to take a few stiff steps forward so that you feel the leg muscles quite tight and stiff. In that tight and stiff leg position, move each leg in a very slow motion in a controlled manner, one leg after the other, just like they do in the military while slow marching. Place each foot firmly on the ground so that you feel the impact and touch of all the toes and the heel.
Carry this exercise as often as it is possible, because it will improve your balance, leg muscles, muscle control, hip/knee/ankle coordination, your upper body balance and coordination, along with mental focus. If you can

reach just to the level that is acceptable to you, you have accomplished a lot.

You do not need to reach a level of excellence, but your efforts will be the greatest reward in many ways. Even in the military, only a few soldiers can achieve excellence in the slow marching. Often during the national day parades around the world, respective armed forces put the best marching soldiers to parade to demonstrate discipline, determination, and will, besides creating an awe, pride, patriotism, inspiration, glory, and confidence among the people. Parades with excellent marching inspire the young men and women to join the military. Therefore, the thought of marching can be a good motivation to good walking. Walking is a healthy habit and all should be addicted to it.

My success record of developing and regaining the BALANCE was very unimpressive. Even though I have been slender, athletic, and active all my life, I experienced great difficulties in regaining my lost balance. After the strokes, I could not walk up and down the stairs without holding on to the handrail and concentrating on my feet during each step I took. It took me more than 5 years to be able to go up and down the stairs without holding handrail. Also, it took me several years to be able to stand on one leg just for one minute. All exercises work differently for each individual, and each individual will take different time periods for recuperation.

There is another very useful exercise for the stroke patient. Patient should open the pantry or kitchen cabinet and insert his or her hand in each shelf freely without touching or striking anything in the process of doing so. Patient should switch from left to right hand after doing it for a couple of times with one hand. Again, the success of the exercise will result only when the patient is able to take each hand, separately, inside the shelves, and take the hand out without touching anything. These and other exercises can be initiated and practiced by the patients themselves without the help of expensive healthcare givers.

If the patients are in position to read the written language, then they should read as often as they can, and try another exercise which will be beneficial for them. Stroke patients should start with reading just a couple of lines in a newspaper or a magazine, and then stop reading. Leave the reading material on the table, and get involved in something else just for a couple of minutes. After this brief break of couple of minutes, the patient should try to recall the content of the written material. Some patients would be successful in remembering what they had read just a few minutes ago, but most may not. This is a completely voluntary exercise on the part of patients who should keep repeating, and once they find themselves remembering the content of just a couple of lines they should go on to larger pieces of written material. This very simple exercise did wonders for my memory which improved considerably over period of time. I could not remember even a few words after reading them, let alone a couple of lines. And now I am writing all this for you, only after several years of practice, and not giving up. Patients do not have to give up anything, and should be on top of everything that is being done to them in any aspect of life. It is easier said than done, but even then do not give up.

Another important exercise is to stimulate the command and movement of the fingers. You know how important the fingers are in the performance of daily functions of life. From a sitting or standing position, place the tip of any one finger of your hand on the table or the arm of the chair. The finger should be in a vertical position and only the finger tip should be touching the flat surface. Now press this finger tip on the flat surface of the table or arm of the chair. Press it, keep it in that position for a few seconds, and then release the pressure. Press it and then release it. Do this a few times every day with each of your fingers. Conduct this exercise everyday. You will develop a considerable strength in your fingers. For the next phase of this exercise, you will be putting all the finger tips of one hand on the flat surface and pressing them all together, and then releasing the pressure. Pressing them, and releasing them. Before you were exercising the fingers individually, and now you are exercising the fingers collectively. In this exercise, just make sure that you use the fingers of one hand at a time. Later, you may choose to use the finger tips of both hands simultaneously.

Let us carry out the exercise of the wrist in conjunction with hand and the fingers. Make a fist and move the fisted hand up, down, left, and right positions. Repeat this exercise a few times with one fisted hand at a time first. Later, you may wish to use both fisted hands together in performing these exercises. Similarly, the forearms and elbows of each arm should be exercised, one arm at a time. Extend one of your arms to its full length, and at this position of your arm form a tight fist. Keep the arm extended. Now bring the tight fist toward your face, by bending the arm at the elbow. This should be done very slowly. Once the fist is closer to your face, then open your hand and let all the fingers spread as much as it is possible. Perform this exercise as often as you can with each arm separately at first. Later, you may wish to use both arms simultaneously. This exercise can be carried out while standing or sitting. The next exercise in this phase is to exercise your shoulders. Drop your hands on your sides, and let them become loose. Now, rotate each arm, one at a time, over your shoulders in an easy way. Rotate as many times as you feel comfortable with. Then do the same kind of rotation with the other arm. After you feel comfortable with one arm rotating at one time, you may rotate both arms simultaneously with ease if you are comfortable with it. These exercises will prove to be good for your circulation in the arms and hands, muscles, bone joints, tendons, movement control, coordination, and upper body in general. Also, after perfecting these exercises, the patients will be able to do basic aerobics.

Focus, attention, memory, strength, and energy happen to be in short supply. Just do one thing at a time, and give yourself a break after a few minutes each time. Doing too many things in a single spell will produce scanty and disheartening results, and therefore will not prove to be encouraging. One task at a time should only be attempted, and once it is complete, then the next task should be undertaken provided there is enough strength and energy left. If not, then wait and rest a while before doing anything else.

All of us need money to survive, and to have money most of us need to work. Work becomes a difficult issue after having even a mild stroke or heart attack. Grown men and women become a highly complex mixture of adults and children, both physically and mentally. It becomes body and brain building and learning process, and the patients and caregivers have got to stay on top of it. If money is not coming in from some source, then the patients have to tap savings or assets to sustain themselves for quite some time. However, life is such that almost all of us, whether under stroke/heart condition or not, end up encountering people with dishonest intentions without fail. Stroke patients have got to be conscious of this, and should guard their money, keep their check books under locks, should stay away from signing any paper received from any one, loved ones and caregivers should make sure that patients do not sign anything without the consent of loved ones, lawyers, doctors, etc. Patient's mind becomes like that of a child, and he or she becomes extremely trusting and credulous. Patients start viewing other people as good and friendly just like children think. Additionally, focus, comprehension, vision, energy, etc. are in extremely short supply with the patients. It would take little or no effort on the part of dishonest people to have stroke patients' signatures on any document. Same thing applies to internet and telephones. In any of such circumstances, patients would not be able to make a correct decision, know the difference between good and bad, compare the issue at hand with something in the past, etc., due to poor or damaged memory, etc. I know this very well. I gave money away, I invested in a small unknown company about which I did not know anything, I sent them substantial amount of money after a few telephone and fax exchanges. This investment company soon went out of business and my investment was lost. My experience with a dentist is almost hair raising, primarily because of my incapacity to make intelligent conversation, analyze, and reason. I gave away my only car to someone I hardly knew. Later, I signed other agreements which turned out to be only in other peoples favor, and I experienced first class exploitation of myself who was stroke patient with very limited vision, energy, weak muscles, weak tendons, little memory, and absolutely no judicious capability. I did not have any loved one, helpful neighbor, care giver. I was doing everything on my own, and exceptional good luck was on my side.

Medical community has come a long way since 1996, and a lot of recognition has been afforded to Stroke. Now, the doctors do listen to you about stroke, and not like before. But still the medical community has yet to catch up similar recognition for women. Women are just as vulnerable to stroke as men. They suffer the same way as men, but somehow whatever attention is given the majority of it goes to men. I remember meeting a newly divorced woman in a party in another city long time ago. She was very beautiful and a picture of femininity which made me think why anyone would want to divorce her. It was during the times when divorcing had started to pick up. We spent time talking and fixed a lunch date. She did not show up, and the whole thing was forgotten. More than a year later, I had signed up for French language class, and the first day I happened to notice someone who looked familiar but was difficult to remember was sitting in the same class. After the class was over, she approached me and apologized for not showing up for the lunch date. Her voice was not clear at all, and her face had changed quite a bit; it was lower on one side than the other. I realized she was the same girl but looked different. Upon asking her as why she was attending French class for beginners when she was fluent in French. She disclosed that she had a stroke, did not know what had happened to her, and various delays took place in providing her the medical help. She was getting better, and needed to go through some basics in French to speed up learning and memory building process. I also learnt from her that her neighbors did not recognize the urgency of sending her to the hospital in time. She went to the hospital on her own after she started to feel bad and helpless. Her conversation revealed that the doctor had the same mind set as that of her neighbors, that is, "nothing is wrong with you," "soon you will be fine", "have some coffee and take a nap". She and many other women were treated as second class citizens when visiting a hospital for a stroke condition.

Today, the medical community is very much aware of the symptoms associated with Stroke. While the knowledge, recognition, care, medicines, etc. are gaining sophistication and advancement, the relative legalities are also becoming very complex. This is primarily due to insurance laws, law suit possibilities, libels, etc. About two years ago, my first cousin had to go through a triple bypass surgery. He had suffered some fainting spells, and he went through a battery of tests, but they all turned out to be normal. After having several additional tests, doctors found out that his heart arteries were clogged, which resulted in triple bypass surgery. Of course, this news made me visit my doctor who ordered Stress Test for me. This was a unique experience for me. My cholesterol, blood pressure, heart beat, pulse beat, and general physical condition were o.k. In the **STRESS TEST**, they wired me with some machines, and I was to spend about 10 minutes on the treadmill. This exercise brought some discomfort on my upper left side of my chest. I passed the test. There were no warning signs found. I was glad when it was over. I felt a strange tiredness with my breathing, and an alarming discomfort on the upper left side between the heart and shoulder blade. Fifteen minutes later at the photocopy shop, I felt dizziness, and I thought I was seconds away from fainting. I drank water, and reached home with some difficulty, where I immediately lay down on the floor and rested for several hours. I felt weak for a several days but got better. I called the nurse and told her what had happened. After a month or two, I was given another type of Test which was similar to the Stress Test except this one had a TV where heart valves could be seen under various levels of stress. While I was on the treadmill, the doctor came and kept me occupied with a lot of conversation and was keeping my eyes away from the treadmill's lever which he was deftly manipulating I was getting tired and uncomfortable, and I told the doctor to stop the treadmill as it was causing stressful fatigue. Doctor kept on going and tilting the treadmill more, and raising the speed. "you are doing fine", "you are in good shape", "another minute won't hurt", etc were the words I heard during this time. I had to shout to have the treadmill stopped because I was feeling very much stressed on the upper left side of my chest, breathing heavily, and I thought I was going to pass out. After he left the room, I was shown the pictures of my heart functioning by the radiologist or assistant. I felt fatigued and aggravated. I asked the radiologist if this test was a leader to bypass surgery, and I followed it by a comment that it was a good surgery marketing program. After a couple of jovial exchanges, he agreed and smiled and acknowledged the fact and said, "There is a lot of money in surgery and money can make people do things" or something like that. I experienced stressful fatigue and tiredness. I passed my stress test completely. I took rest and was back to normal in a few days.

These machine exercises and stress tests may not be suitable for everyone. Every individual is different and comes with different strengths and weaknesses. Those stress tests were not suitable for me and my physical well being. Several months later, I took ultrasound test on my own, and tests showed that clogging in my arteries was much below danger level. This proves that Stress Tests were not good for me, and I could have been the candidate for unnecessary surgery. There could be some other problems with my health but the doctor did not identify them, and I do not feel any different than I should at my age of 67 years. Increased number of legalities will produce more procedures, tests, and formalities, and possibly more surgeries, and definitely no comfort for the patient or the normally healthy persons.

Recently, researchers have discovered that heart related problems can cause stroke. **An estimated 20% Americans have heart defects by birth.** This number may be more in other countries. These defective hearts have small holes in the heart, and the individuals are born with this defect which can cause clots to take formation. These blood clots from the defective hearts, or any other heart condition for that matter, can reach the brain where they can block the blood vessels and cause stroke. Quite often, the medical check ups may produce satisfactory results when, in fact, the health condition of stroke or heart patient may not be satisfactory. The time of the day when the medical test is subjected to a patient is becoming more and more important. Patient's condition could vary at different times of a day. Researchers are becoming aware of various functions of cells in our bodies which regulate insulin, sleep cycles, high and low energy levels, body temperatures, and a host of other things. Tests in one cycle may differ from tests taken during another cycle. It may make the medical treatment more precise in the future, but more complex, difficult, and, therefore, more expensive.

My doctor never prescribed me **ULTRASOUND TEST** of the heart and arteries. But I took these tests on my own without the help of my doctor or the health insurance provider. Life Line Screening conducted these tests on me. The first one was Carotid Artery / Stroke Screening This screening measures the approximate amount of plaque built up in the arteries. It also measures the velocity of blood flow in the arteries. Carotid Arteries are the main sources to transport blood to the brain, and plaque build up in these arteries is the leading cause of stroke. Carotid Arteries run up on the side of the neck, and then branch out in to two arteries. The first one is Internal Carotid Artery which supplies blood to the brain. The second one is the External Carotid Artery which supplies blood to the face and scalp.

The second test that was given to me was Abdominal Aortic Aneurism Screening. Abdominal Aorta Arteries travel from the breast bone to the location of navel, where it branches out in to the Iliac Arteries that supply blood to the legs. Aorta's many branch arteries supply blood to the organs and the abdomen. Ideally Aorta should measure less than 3 centimeters. When it measures 3 centimeters or more, then likelihood of existence of Aneurysm is suspected. There are two kinds of Aneurysm. One is the Fusiform Aneurysm which is when all the walls of Aorta Arteries are enlarged. The other is Saccular Aneurysm which is identified when there is focal enlargement creating a bulge on one side of the Aorta.

The third test was Peripheral Arterial Disease Screening which provides the comparative ratio of blood flow in the arms with the blood flow in the legs. This test is useful to check if you are suffering from Arteriosclerosis. Systolic left arm blood pressure to Systolic left ankle, and Systolic right arm blood pressure to Systolic right ankle are compared.

The fourth test was Osteoporosis Risk analysis, which tests the estimated bone mineral density of the heel bone. Heel bone is similar to the bone found in the spine or hip where most of osteoporosis related fractures occur. Life Line Screening is non invasive, easy, and relatively inexpensive. They have mobile units and travel all over the USA. They can be reached at 1-888-897-9153. Also, similar tests are provided by Healthfair USA who can be reached at 1-888-822-3247.

I cannot forget my dentist's private warning to me. I was advised to be extremely careful since I have graduated to be a senior citizen with Medicare health insurance. I could be taken advantage of by some doctor who needs to perform surgery for one reason or another. Being a senior is not going to be easy for anyone. For the senior citizens power and authority seem to slip away, and the crucial decisions are progressively made by the loved ones and the medical community. If senior citizens suffer stroke or heart attack, their authority is almost diminished, even if the capacity to make decisions remains intact. Decisions end up getting made by loved ones and the doctors. Doctors will protect themselves by ordering just about every kind of test, and on the basis of those tests, they will decide what needs to done with the patient. If surgery is the outcome of their decision, then they will perform surgery. Doctors' personal knowledge, judiciousness, morality, patients' well fair, cost, etc. have, somehow, become secondary. In many parts of world men and women go to the hospital for one kind of ailment, and when they come out, they have one less organ which had nothing to do with the ailment they went to the hospital for. Just think what could happen to a senior citizen. Seniors have Medicare Health Insurance who has lots of money to spend on health services. Also, if the patients happen to be in very bad health condition then they could become organ harvesting candidates, unless they have specific instructions with the medical community to bar them from doing so. Again, loved ones need to be specifically instructed in this regard. Currently, there are 95,000 Americans waiting to receive organs in their bodies and the number is increasing, and you can see the amount of pressure the medical community is under to provide this large number of various organs. To fulfill the demand for organs which is increasing rapidly, the medical community has to find organs that can be transplanted, and these organs happen to be of those near death patients who have agreed to donate them.

A groomed man of around mid 60s nods at me whenever we cross each other in the grocery store. His left foot rises to a very low height, and he raises his right leg way too high in his walk. One day I said hello to him and tried to make some conversation. "I shee yoo often", "warry hot oushide" were the words which told me that he was a stroke patient with speech and movement disability among other (probably). In pursuit of my ego boost, I offered to help him with leg movement, but he declined. His doctor and the healthcare provider controls his well being, and any outside care provider must be approved by healthcare provider and belong to their group. Insurance, contractual legalities, libel, etc. were the issues. I could not understand the complete conversation but I guessed that is what he meant. He was right and seemed like a patient was participating in the process of getting healed. I learned something important that day.

Being a patient does not mean that you have to be in a room whether it is in the hospital or in your home. Go out by yourself, or have someone take you to a public place where people of all walks of life and all ages happen to be present. To get better fast you have to be in the real world where real things are happening, whether you are capable of participating in those activities or not. Try to do this every day, and you will see yourself improving much faster than patients who are in the hospital or home and looking at the same people and the same scene, over and over again.

Point of reference has got to be changed. You cannot afford to sit among other patients day in and day out, and you should not. You will pick up all the disabilities they possess, and they will yours.

You need a complete set of diversified set of reference points, and for this you will have to be in public, and gradually make exchanges. Do not worry about making boo boos that cause humiliations. Just learn to laugh at your own follies; it will do you wonders in getting better. Listen to the language produced by normal people. What you hear, you will produce yourself. If you hear disabled voices continuously, then you will produce the language in the same disabled manner.

> To change the point of reference, I used to make several attempts almost daily to go out of my apartment, and each day over a period of time, I returned with humiliations, failures, and blunders of protocols and decency. But I kept on making efforts to change my environment even just for a few minutes. Several times I had the urge to go away some place where no one knew me and the effect of my strange behavior will be less noticed. After more than 2 years, I gathered enough courage to drive on I-95 south which was to try my relearned driving skills, change the scene, learn things away from home, bring some joy to my life, and test my mettle. My energy levels were good for one hour only. I made every stop there was on I-95 south, including 3 overnight stops, and reached Jacksonville, Florida. The same routine I carried out on my return journey. There were numerous boo boos I made along the way, and I learned from them and corrected them. This proved an important point and that was to stay within the parameters of my energy limits, besides coping with relearning challenges. As long as I remained within these limits I made a lot of progress. It was a great relearning experience and I returned with renewed confidence, stamina, energy, and courage which resulted in my subsequent trips. One aspect of these trips was constant and that was several naps during the day and at least 8 hours of sleep during the night.

> You should determine the parameters of your energy limits, and then attempt something bold every now and then. If you want to drive then I suggest that you familiarize yourself with driving, traffic laws, traffic courtesy, owner's manual, etc. many times again and again, and then start taking very short trips. In the interim, you can take a bus or sit with other drivers and watch others to drive. Also for an outing, take a bus tour and you will be overjoyed with the experience.

Learn something new every day. Just make sure of that, because you want to build up your memory which was lost or partially lost in stroke experience. There is no harm or shame starting at a humble level of such an endeavor. While learning something new every day of the week, please do rerun the previously learned things. Rehashing of any previously learned thing is a super idea, because this exercise instills them deeper in to your memory bank. Regular rehashing will help to remember recently learned things more quickly, and this process will reinforce your confidence in yourself, which means you will be inclined to do better next time around.

As it has been mentioned before, there is no shame in learning, no matter how old you are or how handicapped you may be, and always remember that it's your life, there is limited time in that life span, and you have got to make the best of it. Start with learning something new every day, even if it is something you knew before and you have forgotten it. Be shameless, make errors and learn from them, every day. I do remember my follies and goof ups just about every day. If you wish to try something out of the current realm of capabilities, just go to some other state where no one knows you, and do everything you want to do. If you do something strange, which is likely, the natives will just accept it by saying or concluding that people from your state never knew what they were doing, and that will be it. This goes on in every state where people tend to believe that they are wiser than new arrivals or visitors from other states. It works both ways. They are happy feeling superior, and you get a chance in trying out different things and learning from them.

Shake off the mental DEPRESSION. It is a process which requires some patience. When we feel helpless, cornered, unloved, disconnected, sleepless, stressed, tired, defeated, with low self esteem, etc., we develop a depressed state of mind. This depressed state of mind at first is just temporary, or a passing phase, like a bad day at work, or a bad weather day. But if it persists for quite some time, then this depressed state of mind causes chemical imbalance in the brain. From emotional problem the depression has become physiological also. What a negative addition to the patient's state of health. Doctors have medication to stabilize this chemical imbalance, which does provide a relief to the patients. These medications, when used over a period of time, may make the patients dependent on them. Just how many medications you have appetite for and money for to buy them? If uncontrolled, most of our day planner could be filled with pill popping times. If medication has been prescribed by the physician, then do take it, but don't stop thinking about getting better at the same time without your own personal efforts. You have to get better, and getting better cannot be and should not be outsourced exclusively to some medical institution, just because you have healthcare plan and you regularly contribute to it. Contribute to your healthcare plan regularly but try to use it sparingly. Self participation in the healing process and controlling it will contribute greatly to speed up the recovery process. Sustained high stress levels can contribute to a variety of health problems.

First of all it is important to know that sadness, tension, frustration, mistakes, inability to function properly and control activities, etc. can cause STRESS. Stress can disrupt or reduce the flow of blood to the brain and heart, because under stressful state the blood vessels constrict which results in disruption of normal blood flow. It also raises the blood pressure to a higher level. If stress remains unchecked or uncontrolled, then another Stroke or Heart Attack can occur. You already know that the medical professionals give you a number of tests to predict the probability of stroke or heart attack occurrence. Unfortunately, the medical professionals never subject the patients to an **EMOTIONAL TEST** which, in fact, is equally important if not more, because stress levels are directly dependent on emotional state of any person.

Although I recognize the fact that there is some degree of stress in our daily life, but to let it go unchecked and ignore it will definitely prove to be a folly. Before we can CURE stress, we need to micro analyze it to find the root causes which are affecting our thinking and life in general. Somehow, we tend to expend a lot of emotional energy on various stress causing problems, because we often do not know the root cause, or the possible acceptable solution. Once we go through the process of analyzing causes of stress, we reach a specific understanding on individual basis. Each individual is different with different personality, reasons for stress, degrees of stress levels etc. and, therefore, requires specific measures to reduce stress. Here are some general suggestions based on my own experience at different times.

To relieve yourself from stress, or to minimize it, breathe deeply as often as it is comfortable for you. While deep breathing, the patient should concentrate on the breathing itself. Do this deep breathing as many times a day as you comfortably can, and it will help you. Think of how green your valley was. Think of the old good days when everything was clicking without any problems whatsoever. Reminisce the exhilarating past events and experiences which provided you with joy and hope for the future. Think of all the people you like and whose company you enjoy the most, revisit the conversations and jokes you shared together. Think of the person you loved the most in your life, Visualize the faces of people who like you no matter what circumstances you happen to be in. Also, visualize the people who would like to be in your company. Be optimistic, no matter how bad the circumstances may be. Optimistic people are considered to be generally successful and happy in life, because they carry hope for the future. Think that the problems at hand will pass through one day, and all will become normal once again. Usually, this is the case which has happened to me many times in my life. Think of some past funny incidents and enjoy the details rerunning them in your mind. Think of some jokes you heard in the past and enjoyed them. Watch cartoons on TV. Watch comedy channel on TV. Read books of jokes. Get involved in some indoor or outdoor game and/or sport. Walk a little to change the scene, Shoot some breeze with some one sitting on the next table while having coffee. etc. Most importantly, learn to verbalize your stressful problems, learn to reflect on important issues of life, and also learn to introspect, which will prove to be very constructive in the long run.

Medical community knows that insufficient quantities of Serotonin in the brain can lead people to the state of DEPRESSION. Without Serotonin, or in insufficient quantities of Serotonin in the brain, patients' will feel depression. In a normal brain, the blood flows normally and evenly in the brain, however, in a depressed patient's brain, blood flows irregularly and there are several spots where blood supply is completely absent or at a minimum level. Serotonin is believed to be found in omega-3 fatty acids which are found in certain kinds of fish, or in the form of fish oil capsule. Certain prescribed doses of fish oil with omega-3 have been known to increase the amount of Serotonin in the frontal cortex of brain. Eskimos, especially of Greenland, do not suffer from depression because most of their diet is fish which contains Serotonin. Depressed people have low levels of omega-3 in their blood. But moderation comes to play here once again. There are two families of fatty acids which are essential for the body. Omega-6 and Omega-3. Omega-6 lowers and controls the blood cholesterol, and is inflammatory. Omega-3 cleans the inside walls of the arteries and is non-inflammatory. Both are good and cannot be inter-changed. Both need to be consumed in an optimal ratio to each other. Very high levels of omega-6 may not be beneficial to most people. Arachidonic acid (AA) is found in Omega-6, which tend to cling to the inside of arterial walls and causes blockage of the blood vessels, and is among the reasons of causing inflammation. Eicosapentaenoic is a part of Omega-3, and tend to clean the inside of arterial walls, and is non-inflammatory. The ratio of Arachidonic acid (AA) and Eicosapentaenoic acid (EPA) must be at an optimal level for a healthy body. AA/EPA ratio is high among depressed people.

Omega 6 and Omega-3 are essential to the body. They are important components of cell membranes to maintain flexibility and to keep it fluid. They are the building blocks of chemical messengers, known as Prostaglandins, that regulate cardio vascular function, brain, nervous system, fat, and metabolism, flexibility of joints, skin health, and protective response to any inflammation. Important sources of Omega-3 are: fish like mackerel, herring, sardines, tuna, sturgeon, anchovy, sprat, cod level, flax seed, walnuts, hemp seeds. Prominent sources of Omega-6 are oils like: olive oil, canola oil, corn oil, peanut oil, flax seeds/oil, black current oil, borage oil, and primrose oil. Balance and moderation are keys to consuming them for your good health. You can also derive Omega-6 and Omega-3 fatty acids from a vegetarian diet source. Both, Omega-6 and Omega-3, are found with varying ratios to each other in soy beans, tofu, soy milk, berries, peas, beans, and the oils of flax seeds, walnuts, canola (rape seed), soy, and so forth. Omega 6 reduces HDL (good) cholesterol, promotes blood clotting, increases blood pressure, and increases oxidation of LDL (bad) cholesterol. On the other hand, Omega 3 lowers triglycerides (3 fatty acids), reduces the chances of sudden cardiac death, and decreases the sub class of small particles of LDL (bad) cholesterol. Also, Omega 3 is anti clotting, anti diabetic, lowers lipoprotein, anti depressant, and reduces the chances of inflammation in the coronary plaque. Triglycerides are large molecules of fatty substance. This is the fat which is stored in the body, and it does not contain cholesterol. This fat gets accumulated in the body through diet of various vegetable and animal fats and carbohydrates in our food intake. Limited fat is good for our body, but it should be around 10% and no more. People with high triglycerides have lower HDL (good cholesterol) and higher levels of LDL (bad cholesterol). Lower the triglycerides the better it is. Omega 3 lowers triglycerides.

DEPRESSION is caused by nutritional deficiency, especially vitamin B, stress induced vitamin deficiency, heavy metal toxicity, mercury, cadmium, lead, artificial food additives, too much coffee, unnecessary drugs, occupational toxins, etc. Also, a sudden drop in the sugar level in the blood can cause lethargy and depression.

Depressed people have low levels of omega-3 in their blood stream. We already know that AA is inflammatory. Here is a simple way to compare the two fatty acids:

Omega-6 fatty acids are inflammatory, while omega-3 fatty acids are anti-inflammatory. Both are essential fatty acids for a healthy body. The ideal ratio of AA/EPA, or Omega-6 to Omega-3, is 3:1. (3gram of Omega-6, to 1gram of Omega-3). Variables are dependent upon the severity of depression, body weight, ethnicity, age, etc. Dr. Floyd Chilton and

Laura Tucker explain in The Inflammation Nation that Omega 6 to Omega 3 ratio of 3:1 is adequate to reduce inflammation in the arteries and therefore may reduce the incidence of cardio vascular disease.

Mind can play tricks on the body. DEPRESSION can adversely influence the immune system of the body, which can result in a host of problems with stomach and nervous system. To get rid of depression, first of all start WALKIING. You do not need special clothing or shoes for walking. Start walking in your house, apartment, or in your own private room. Keep on walking as long as you like it, or for as long as long as you can comfortably. Walk as if this is the only thing you know how to do, and this is the only purpose you have got at the moment in life. Walk from your kitchen to your bathroom via the bedroom, and keep on repeating this circle aimlessly. If you are using a walker, then do this routine with walker. Your walking may be similar to that of a person who has nothing to do any given day and walking is the only thing to pass the time with. TV can be a distraction. Use as many different shoes as you may have to conduct your walking routine. Changing shoes will provide you stimulation in almost all the muscles in your legs, and feet. Also, different shoes have different characteristics in design, shape, materials, etc. which will stimulate slightly different regions of your leg muscles and feet.

During this walking time, let your mind wander from one thing to another. Let it go freely wherever it takes you. Your thoughts may take you to the burnt toast for breakfast, the smelly caregiver, not enough light, doctor spoke too fast for you to remember anything, relatives did not bring any gifts during their recent visit, what a great song that was, that was a great humor, enjoyable company, delicious dinner, great movie and great theme, someone brought you a bouquet of flowers which seemed old and withered, coffee was no where hot, children had a good time, how to make my spouse bring some decent snacks, how to get some private moments with loved one, etc. Soon, you will graduate from this kind of walking, and venture out to the courtyard or a park where you have much more room to do the same kind of walking and thinking. Very soon, but definitely soon, you will feel much better at the end of the day. Beneficial results will appear in various areas with varied degrees.

FALLING is a serious danger we all face, whether we are a patient or not. If you happen to be a stroke or heart attack patient, then your energy, strength, and focus levels are on the low par level, and there should be extra care in this regard. Safeguard yourself by having skid proof rugs, bathtub mats, bathtub hand grab bars and hand rails, well lit rooms and hall ways, climb up or down the stairs with human help, try to stay on the same floor for all activities, and try to see that all the needed things to live are within easy grab.

BREATHING plays an important role in shaking off DEPRESSION Breathing is the mechanism to sustain life even just for a minute. Breathing is essential to living. The operation of brain and the nervous system is basically dependent upon oxygen and carbon dioxide exchange. Oxygen in and carbon dioxide out are crucial for life. Correct way to breath is therapeutic, and can ward off many diseases as well. Correct breathing is when we involve our stomachs in the breathing process. Most of us have been taught that breathing involves lungs only. However, when we breathe in a way that our stomach inflates and deflates with each breath in and out, we are not only involving lungs but also the stomach. This method is relaxing. Your belt and clothing around the belly and chest should be loose. Try to concentrate on each breath you take, and also try to listen to the sound of your breathing-in and out. You will be surprised to find it to be extremely relaxing; it is good for our body and it is good for our brain. This exercise will supply oxygen to organs and the brain with the help of oxygen rich blood. If you wish to take this breathing habit to the next level, then try this one. Lie down on any flat surface, preferably on the floor carpet. Lie straight, face up looking at the ceiling. Now start breathing in this manner, and focus on your breathing. Focus on breathing is important. You will see that when you breathe through the stomach, your stomach will inflate and deflate. Breathing in this posture will give you more relaxation than in sitting position. This posture of lying flat on your back, and breathing through your stomach is a great sleep inducing. Depressed people find it hard to sleep, and this breathing method could improve quality and duration of sleep. If this aspect of life is rectified and achieved, then a major accomplishment in shaking off depression has been realized.

LAUGHTER has been known as the best cure for most ailments, and there is no doubt about it. Laughter is a great stress reliever. You should stimulate laughter through humor which is also good for positive mental activity and engagement. Other stress relieving outlets are speaking with a lot of people if possible, getting involved in pleasurable activities, developing new and old relationships (openly and privately), getting involved in serious love affairs if you are single, visiting an inspirational place of your liking, adopting a pet, doing good deeds for others, deep breathing, dreaming and fantasizing, visualizing that you are completely recovered and are in very good health, music, Yoga, Tai Chi, etc. In doing and accomplishing process, we must realize one thing that whatever we do and for whatever purpose we do it, that becomes a physical part of our brains, and we end up living with it for the rest of our life. All the things we think, promise, do, emotions we extend, and emotions we receive, etc. become a part of our life that we will be living. There is no escape from this reality. Therefore, it becomes imperative that whatever we think and do must be the things that we are willing to live with happily, and not regretfully. If we end up doing something contrary to this, we have sewn the seeds for stress in our own brain, and these seeds will find company with other controversial seeds whether subjectively sewn or brought in from outside through interactions with people. The combination of these contradictions will accumulate over time and will eventually bring us a stroke or heart attack experience or some other equally deadly health condition.

NATURE provides everything inside the body and outside for the sustenance and cure of our bodies. Vegetables, fat free yogurt, fruits, grains, olive oil, fresh water fish are some of the good things, among many other, that stroke patients and all others should consume on a regular basis. Of course, stroke patients require foods that are good for the brain for the obvious reasons to get well faster in a sustaining manner. The most important food items that would cover this healing category are:

Olive oil, onions, garlic, thyme, parsley, rosemary, basal, soy products, green, beans, potatoes, green and red peppers, egg plant, lemon and lime juice, pasta, mushrooms, tomatoes and tomato sauce, rice, celery, carrots, green peas and dried peas, Lima and northern beans, turmeric, cumin, and parsley.

Of course, you must emphatically inform your doctor about what you eat every day. Doctors seldom ask the patient about their daily diet and the ingredients. Most of the time, they just tell you vaguely what to eat and what to avoid.

Medical community prescribes anti-coagulants to the stroke and heart patients, to save their life by deterring further strokes or heart attacks which are caused by clogged or blocked arteries. Anti-coagulants thin the blood so that it can easily pass through the clogged or blocked areas of arteries. Nature provides this anti-coagulant, the blood thinner, in the form of vitamin K. Vitamin K is found in the following mentioned foods:

Asparagus, avocados, beans, broccoli, cabbage, Brussels sprouts, cauliflower, Cole slaw, collard greens, unpeeled cucumbers, endives, chick peas, scallions, kale, lentils, lettuce, liver (beef, pork, chicken), raw mustard greens, parsley, green peas, dill pickles, sauerkraut, sea weed, soy bean, spinach, swiss chard, turnip greens, water cress

Other foods that contain some vitamin K are:

Canola oil, soybean oil, mayonnaise, margarine, alcoholic drinks, green tea, sweet cloves tea, danshen, devils claw, dong quai, papain

These foods are natural blood thinners. If you are visiting the doctor for a stroke or heart related condition, then you must talk about this with your doctor without fail. Generally, the doctors prescribe anti-coagulants to patients, so it is imperative that the stroke or heart patient advises the doctor that some of the above mentioned foods are being consumed. This will help and remind the doctor to adequately prescribe the medicine for the patient. If, for example, your daily food contains ample amount of iron or calcium, and you happen to take additional supplements in the form of vitamins and minerals (in tablet form) then, perhaps, you are overloading your physical system with nutrients, and may suffer health related repercussions later. Prescribing doctor must be told of the contents and the amount of foods you consume each day. On the other hand, if for any reason, combination of food, medicines, and vitamin supplements do not make real sense to you, then make sure that you do not delay in discussing this specific feeling with your doctor, or any other doctor, read upon it, write to researchers and institutions, explore the internet for similar information, etc. Just do not sit on it and do nothing. It is your body, and you have to feel responsible for its well being.

More than a year ago, upon the advice of my doctor, I started to take high potency calcium tablets each day, because I learned that high doses of calcium could prevent **OSTEOPOROSIS** which, in common language, is described as loss of bone density which leads to shrinkage of bone mass, loss of height, bones without elasticity, brittle bones which can break easily. Just after 10 days of taking supplemental calcium tablets, I started to feel pain in my back just below the rib cage. The pain was similar to muscle sore or light sprain after a fatiguing exercise routine. After suffering for several days, I started to believe that the pain was coming from blocked kidneys. Repeated use of muscle rub did not make the pain go away. One afternoon, I found myself unable to breathe comfortably and I felt dizzy. I sensed that I was about to get very sick with some serious health problem related to heart, head, or some thing else, so I wanted to get out of my apartment confines and reach the hall way where some neighbor could see me and call the ambulance. But I just succeeded to reach the front door, reached for the door handle but could not open it because I collapsed and was completely out of myself. After about one and half hours I came to my senses and realized that I was lying crouched up on the little shoe rubbing carpet just at the entrance, and I despised myself finding myself lying there. I got up; the pain was still in my back. I felt lucky and thanked God for my being able to get revived. In condo apartments, no one enters your premise, and unless you have some kith and kin no one would even bother to inquire. In this case, I could have died and neighbors would not have known until the foul smell of the decaying body had entered the hallway. I took several glasses of water and rested, and analyzed and reasoned out the proximate cause of such an occurrence. It turned out to be that calcium supplement was the only new thing in my diet. So, I stopped taking it and flushed my kidneys with lot of water among other liquids. The pain went away. Now, it has been more than a year. Even after gardening for 4 to 5 hours, I never experienced pain in my back. I was fortunate to link calcium supplement to back pain. This problem could have stemmed from something entirely different reason as well.

There is a lot of emphasis over liquids in our body. At the same time, there seems to be a kind of passion to drink bottled **WATER**. In fact, it has become a kind of health fad and fashion to be seen drinking from a bottled water. Also, production of bottled water has increased several folds to meet the market demands. It is no longer customary to offer someone a drink of tap water which is scoffed at. I never switched to bottled water. I drink it only when I am traveling when tap water is not readily available. I think the government agencies take care of the quality of water they provide to the public. In this case, I trust the government more than private enterprises. Bottled water may lack important minerals which are essential for our body. Bottled water may not contain calcium, magnesium, and fluoride, and if certain brands do then they are at very low levels. There may be some water bottling plant that does provide these essential minerals in their product, but I am not aware of it. So, do consider this aspect of bottled water, before depending on it. Tap water is as good as the water can be, and if there is any doubt in your mind then boil it and cool it before drinking it.

This takes us to various nutritional supplements, and their health related beneficial or not so beneficial affects. So, just be careful when you consume nutritional food with supplements. Over doing in any nourishing ingredient could be laying out foundation for some other ailment in the near future.

The VITAMIN and MINERAL supplements that we consume daily are important source of nutrition, no doubt, because they provide our body with nutrition that is lacking in our daily food intake. If, for any reason and without being aware of it, we happen to take same vitamin supplements that are abundantly found in our daily food in take, then we are definitely overloading our bodies with certain nutrients, whether they happen to be vitamins, minerals, or metals. All sorts of physical complications can emerge as a result of such overloading. So, discuss such matters with your doctor, friends, and read upon it on a regular basis.

Lately, a lot of recognition to stroke and heart related condition has been given by the medical research community. In recent years, Trans Fatty Acids, sub-strata of LDL, was identified as major culprit in causing stroke and heart attacks. Some Trans fatty acids occur naturally in our body; however, the man made ones are the dangerous ones. Liquid vegetable oils, such as soybean and cottonseed oils, were engineered to replace as healthier alternatives to animal fats. These vegetable oils are bombarded with hydrogen atoms in a complex process which is commonly known as Partial Hydrogenation. The end result was stiffer and stable fat which increased the shelf life of manufactured foods. This instigated a switch from butter to margarine. Margarine became very popular with food manufacturers. For example, crackers made with this stiffer fat can remain crispy on the shelf for several years. As of January 1, 2006, FDA requires all food labels to list the amount of Trans Fat in the food.

ARACHIDONIC ACIDS, commonly known as AA are one of the major building blocks for Inflammatory messengers. When we get a paper cut, the area of cut swells and become red. Prostaglandins (messengers) encourage the surrounding blood vessels to dilate, so that it becomes easier for the army of white blood cells to get in. Blood when rushing out produces redness and swelling, this is inflammation. Prostaglandins stimulate nerves to send out pain messages to the brain. Pain is the message which tells you to stop whatever you are doing. Without pain, we will not take our hands off a hot surface. Commonly used pain killers like aspirin, Advil, etc, when ingested, tend to reduce the production of **PROSTAGLANDINS**. These medicines are designed to block the production itself.

LEUKOTRIENES are another kind of inflammation messenger, which helps to direct the army of white blood cells in an entirely different way. These leukotrienes messengers direct the army of white blood cells to the exact locations with messages of degree of intensity. The amount of leukotrienes present at the scene of white cell attack is proportionate to the scale of attack. Just like in war, specific number of soldiers equipped with specifically suitable fighting gear for a specific target is dispatched. When the normal inflammation process to save the site of injury and the body tissue becomes abnormal, then it becomes dangerous for the body.

INFLAMMATION disease is primarily due to too much of good things that are happening in side the body. Red alert do save our bodies. But when the internal dial is set on red alert permanently, then it becomes dangerous for the body. It can occur through miscalculation on the part of our body by sending too many messengers to defend a specific site in the body, when there is no need to do so. Emergency crew is dispatched continuously to the site to find no emergency each and every time. Too many rescue squads are dispatched when there is no disaster. This causes a tremendous jolt and damage to the body tissue which in turn results in inflammation. This process is painful and destructive for the body.

When our body produces higher quantities of prostaglandins, it makes for blood vessels to dilate, which results in more redness and swelling. More prostaglandins mean more pain. This results in more leukotrienes and therefore more white cells are dispatched. More damage is resulted. This is our body's natural healing and protective process. If it gets out of whack, then it causes serious damage to the body. Just imagine what happens when such dispatches of white cell army are sent to any part of our brain.

Inflammation in any part of our body, especially in our brain or heart can be devastating. Many researchers and Dr. Chilton theorize that inflammation plays a key role in the development and progression of atherosclerosis, besides in asthma, various allergies, rheumatoid arthritis, diabetes, chronic kidney failure, chronic hepatitis, chronic thyroid disease, chronic pancreatitis, arthritis, chronic bronchitis, emphysema, Alzheimer's dementia, cancer.

Medical community knows that over supply of inflammatory messengers plays the most prominent role in the Inflammation Disease. It is also known that our body produces these Inflammatory Messengers from fatty acids known as Arachidonic Acids (AA). High levels of Arachidonic Acids (AA) cause over production of Inflammatory Messengers. Therefore, we must control the amount of AA in our blood. Just to acknowledge the presence of AA in our daily food in take, we see the following 5 categories as described by Dr. Floyd Chilton and Laura Tucker

INFLAMMATORY INDEX
(index value/100g of serving)

Egg yolk		340/100g
Turkey Dark Meat		160/100g
Chicken Dark Meat		100/100g
Pork Chops		50/100g
Lamb Loin		70/100g
Beef Hamburger	(95% lean)	40/100g

According to Dr. Chilton, the total daily consumption of foods with AA/EPA index should be less than 150

High proportions of trans fatty acids (AA) are found naturally and in hydrogenated unsaturated oils. Disproportionate amounts of Trans fatty acids (AA) inhibit an essential enzyme that is produced by the liver to convert cholesterol in to BILE acids. Bile acids are the vehicle to transport cholesterol out of the body. If, on the other hand, cholesterol is not converted to bile acids, then cholesterol accumulates in the blood.

Balance is the key word in the total food we consume on regular basis. This includes dairy, meats, poultry, sea food, vegetables, grains, nuts, oils, minerals, vitamins, metals, alcohol, coffee, tea, etc. The concerned people should give consideration to the following mentioned when assessing their intake of certain nutrients:

SATURATED FATS: These fats increase cholesterol in the blood stream. These fats are usually solid at room temperature. Some prominent sources of these fats are:
Hard cheeses, butter, ice cream, cream, sour cream, cream cheese, cocoa butter, chocolate, meats, organs, processed meats, beef, pork, chicken, whole fat dairy products, whole milk, regular yogurt, liver, kidneys, hot dogs, cold cuts, palm/coconut/palm kernel oils.

MONOUNSATURATED FATS: These fats decrease blood cholesterol. These fats are liquid at room temperature. Amazingly, these fats have no effect on High Density Lipoproteins (HDL), also known as the good cholesterol. Monounsaturated fats are found in:
Olive, canola, and peanut oils, olives, avocados, peanuts, almonds, cashews, pistachios, pecans, brazil nuts, fatty vegetables, etc.

PLOYUNSTURATED FATS: These fats are also cholesterol lowering fats provided consumed in combination with low fat diet. They are liquid at room temperature. They may lower the levels of good cholesterol (HDL) if consumed in large quantities. They are found in soy nuts, chestnuts, walnuts; sunflower, corn, soybean, sesame, cotton seed, safflower oils, sunflower seeds, sesame, pumpkin seeds.

CHAPTER VI

SIMPLE PRECAUTIONS

AVOID THE SECOND OCCURRENCE OF STROKE OR HEART ATTACK

We want to avoid having a Stroke or a heart attack. If we have had one then we do not want to have another one, and overall we want to get better, and stay in good health. To avoid having a stroke or recognizing the initial symptoms of coming stroke, then we must recognize the signals associated with it. An experience where no reason exists, or an experience of sudden sensation which describes, or comes close to it, the following scenario: Sudden severe headache without a cause and sometime it is very painful beyond expression, a sudden drop in the vision with a feeling that eyesight has diminished and diminishing even further, both cheeks and the face do not feel comfortable when touched, there is some kind of lifelessness or numbness in the leg, arm, face and other places; loss of balance, walking difficulties, dizziness, difficulty in speaking and understanding, dropped energy levels, feeling related to sagging body, and a variety of confusion should be of alarm. The on set of heart attack will produce chest pains, breathing difficulties, flushed and somewhat swollen face, dizziness, feeling of vomiting, consistent back pain emanating from the point just below the left shoulder blade, traveling pain from the chest to the neck and to left arm, and then affecting other parts of the body.

If such a scenario presents itself to you or anyone you know, man or women, just call 911 right away. After calling 911, take one aspirin with a full glass of water, and sit in a comfortable position or lie down. Talking, questions and answers, TV, etc. would not be good for the patients well being, so just avoid that before and after the ambulance arrives. Patient will recover if quietness, rest, cooperation, no aggravation, medical help are afforded to him or her without delay. We, as patients or care givers, must remind ourselves that when we happen to be on Stroke or heart attack scene, our each action can stimulate the process of life saving or disability and death for the patient. So we must be very careful even if we have all the good wishes for the patient. Over zealous or over active minded well wishers can surely speed up the patient's journey to the grave. Often the patient can heal depending on various other factors, without much medical help, and thereafter resume a normal life in a gradual manner. In this process and in any other process of healing the Patient is the star of playing the major role by initiating and actively participating in the healing process for himself or herself.

REMOVING TOXINS FROM THE BLOOD

Over the years, people have known that clean blood means good health. Chemicals, toxins, excessive fat, calcium, plaque, excessive minerals and metals, etc. block the flow of blood. Chelation therapy is believed to reduce calcium and plaque lodged on the arterial walls. The atherosclerotic plaque can occur in any artery of the body, and is not limited to the arteries near the brain or heart. This plaque can stop or reduce the flow of blood. Blood carries oxygen to various parts of the body. Lack of oxygen results in death of cells. It is believed that there are over 75,000 miles of blood vessels in our body, largest ones to the smallest ones, which supply blood to every cell tissue, gland, and organ in the body. In an adult body, there is about one liter of blood for every 25 lbs of body weight. There are red blood cells and white blood cells in our body. Red blood cells are smaller cells, and in fact they are much smaller than other body cells as well. It is estimated that there are about 25,000,000,000,000 red blood cells in our body, and each one lasts for just 100 days after which they are destroyed by the body. This means that every second about 3 million of red cells are being removed and replaced. Each one of these red blood cells contains about 300 million hemoglobin molecules. And each of these haemoglobin molecules can capture and carry four molecules of oxygen. This means that about 1,000 million molecules of oxygen are transported by each cell as it circulates through the lungs. In a sitting position, the heart beat is normal, and it sends out oxygen rich blood to the body without resting. With each heart beat, 500,000,000,000,000,000,000,000 oxygen molecules are carried out by hemoglobin molecules. If for some reason, the breathing stops, it will mean that the consistent supply of oxygen molecules has been cut off. Supply of oxygen is critical for the brain to survive and function, and there are not more than 3 or 4 minute supply of oxygen reserve in the body at any given time. Supply of oxygen to the brain is so critical that it can best be exemplified by saying that if the carotid arteries which pass through the sides of the neck to the brain are squeezed tight, unconsciousness will result within seconds. Hemoglobin molecules carry oxygen, sugars, and amino acids, etc. to the brain, but oxygen has the most critical place in all of them. From time to time, a blood cell count is necessary and good for the stroke and heart patients, and the doctors should make sure that they maintain accurate records on each patient. Each patient is different, and their individual normal blood count may differ from others,

We have talked about **OXYGEN** a few times, and we know that without it we cannot survive for more than just a couple of minutes. We also know that when cells in various parts of our body do not receive oxygen through uninterrupted flow of blood, they just die. If many cells die in a particular part of the body, then that part also dies or become limp and half dead. Of course, we do not carry oxygen canisters wherever we go, we just breathe in the oxygen that is available through the air. How many of us are really aware of the oxygen content of the air in our house or apartment? We take oxygen for granted, because wherever we are we can breathe freely. We never pause to think if the air we are breathing has sufficient amount of oxygen or not, and that is in your house or apartment. We breathe where we work and live. Ironically, the oxygen content of most work places and living quarters is much less than we would desire to have, especially in comparison to the outside air. In the cold climate where heating and air conditioning are mostly used to make the inside temperature somewhat comfortable during winter and summer seasons, we hardly open the doors and windows to let the fresh air come in. If we do decide to open the doors and window during these two seasons then we are inviting higher energy cost which has never been anyone's first preference. It has been known that the oxygen content of air in any such work place or living quarter is at a much lower level than we think. It is an unhealthy environment. Additionally, various bacteria can live and thrive for several generations in these closed and protected quarters where temperature is controlled almost year around. If possible, then please do relate this environmental condition to various ailments that keep repeating from time to time. This is a good reason to get out of your room, no matter for how short a period that might turn out to be. Do get out as often as you can. Going out will let you breathe fresh air which has much more oxygen than is available in your home or office.

CHELATING THERAPY is intra venous as well as oral. Intravenous, involves injecting chelating agents in to the blood stream to eliminate undesirable substances like heavy metal, chemicals, toxins, mineral deposits and fatty plaques. In this therapy process, EDTA (Ethylene, Diamien Tetra acetic Acid) is injected in the blood stream. Chelating agents (EDTA) are substances which can chemically bond with metals, minerals, chemical toxins, etc. In fact these agents encircle the ions of metals, minerals, chemicals, toxins, and carry them out of the body via urine and feces. Organic acids naturally found in our bodies and in foods can act as Chelating agents, including acetic acid, ascorbic acid (vitamin C), citric and lactic acids. Natural chelating process allows us to experience digestion, assimilation and transportation of food nutrients, along with the formation of enzymes, and hormones, and detoxification of toxic chemicals and metals. Nature does it all by itself. Oral Chelating therapy is much slower than intravenous. Dr. Gary Gordon, co founder of American College of Advancement in Medicine and a pioneer in Chelating therapy, believes that chelating agents will be able to save millions of lives each year in the United States alone.

Chelating therapy with EDTA was first introduced in the USA in 1948 as a treatment for LEAD Poisoning, Workers were found to have lead poisoning caused by the environment in the Battery Factory where they worked. Later Naval Sailors were treated for lead poisoning for having subjected to painting the ships and other facilities. Physicians who were treating these workers in the battery factory and naval sailors who were painting ships, with chelating therapy, were surprised that patients who also had Atherosclerosis (fatty plaque built up in the arterial walls) or Arteriosclerosis (hardening of the arteries) experienced reduction in both conditions. Chelating therapy with EDTA has been reportedly successful with numerous beneficial effects.

Some of reported benefits have been reduction in blood clumping and preventing blood clots, marked improvement in patients with vascular diseases, improved cognitive function in people with memory and concentration deficits, improved visual acuity (specially when problem caused by arterial blockages), reduction of blood fat levels, improved and increased blood flow to extremities of the body, decalcification of elastic tissue resulting in improved elasticity and resilience, decreased blood pressure levels, various levels of benefits for aneurysm, Alzheimer, senile dementia, arthritis, diabetes, osteoporosis, Parkinson disease, varicose veins, stroke, venomous snake bites, etc.

Amazingly, 90% of Americans face danger from illness related to blood circulatory system. The treatment of CVD alone costs more than $ 1 Billion annually.

$200,000 every minute An estimated cost of a bypass surgery is $400,000 per case. Inter venous Chelating therapy is far less invasive and expense driven. But there is one danger associated with Chelating therapy which may lower the levels of calcium in the bones and teeth. To replace the calcium drawn from the blood by Chelating therapy with EDTA, body will draw calcium from bones and teeth to replace it. A thorough testing and approval by your personal physician will be required before undertaking such a therapy.

Oral chelation that is when nutritious food supplements in combination with certain chelating agents, like EDTA ad other natural chelaters, including vitamins, minerals, amino acids, antioxidants, and herbs are taken on a scheduled basis, is quite affective. In spite of the fact that it is a much slower method but it will accomplish the same as intra venous chelating would. It is believed to reduce heavy metal toxicity and calcification, it will lower cholesterol, it will reduce free radical oxidation of metabolized fats, it will prevent formation of blood clots, etc

AVOID CONSUMING TOXINS

Stroke and heart patients should avoid consuming, or minimize the consumption of canned vegetables, butter, baking soda, alcohol, caffeinated drinks, mold prohibitors, preservatives, tenderizers, artificial sweeteners, commercially prepared foods, chlorinated tap water, fats from commercially raised animals, fast food oils, hydrogenated or partially hydrogenated oils, lard, margarine, mono sodium glutamate, processed and refined foods and meats, soft drinks, softened tap water, sugars, and fast foods, trans fatty acids, tallow tropical oils, white flour foods

CARDIO VASCULAR HEALTH

Deficiencies of certain nutrients in the body can cause Cardio Vascular Disease (CVD). Some vitamins and minerals are vital for a healthy cardio vascular system. Vitamins C, E, A, D, B, including beta carotene, niacin, niacinamide, folic acid, and biotin are supposed to be essential for CV health. Among minerals, calcium, chromium, copper, magnesium, manganese, molybdenum, potassium, selenium and zinc stand out to be the important ones. Amino acids like carnitine, lysine, praline, and coenzyme Q-10 have been strongly recommended. Some of these nutrients may protect you against heavy metal absorption and toxicity. You may take magnesium to ward off the ill affects of aluminum. To avoid ill affects of arsenic in your body, try taking amino acids with sulfur, calcium, iodine, selenium, vitamin C, and zinc. Cadmium absorption can be minimized by taking amino acids with sulfur, calcium, vitamin C, and zinc. Absorption of lead in the body can be minimized by taking amino acids including sulfur, pectin (alginate), selenium, vitamin C, There are several oral chelating formulas developed by medical professionals over the years, with primarily one objective and that is to remove metals and toxins from the body.

METALS IN OUR BODY

Metals and toxins can be extremely hazardous to stroke patients and completely healthy people as well. Metals and toxins tend to clog the blood vessels in one way or another. More importantly, metals damage the arterial walls, causing ruptures, inflammation and blood clotting, and blocking or minimizing the flow of blood to the brain. Here is a brief description of each metal which is not only hazardous to the brain but other parts of the body as well.

We get **ALUMINUM** in our bodies from cookware, baking powder, aluminum foil, salad dressings, pickles, some ready to serve grated parmesan cheese, some table salts, anti-acids, antiperspirants, various feminine hygiene products, buffered aspirin, canned acidic foods, food additives, lipstick, drugs, medications, processed cheese, softened water, and tap water. Aluminum targets bones, brains, kidneys, and stomach. Kidney damage, liver dysfunction, loss of appetite, loss of balance, muscle pain, shortness of breath and weakness may signal excess of aluminum in the body. Aluminum causes, neurological disorders like: Alzheimer's disease, Parkinson's disease, senile and pre-senile dementia, staggering while walking, inability to pronounce words properly, memory loss, difficulties in behavior among children in school, etc. Aluminum gets in to the water through acid rain. Industrial smoke stacks cause release of sulfur in to the atmosphere, which falls back to earth's surface in the form of sulfuric acid. Sulfuric acid kills fish, vegetable life, and threatens humans. Sulfuric acid reacts with various substances in the soil, and turns them in to aluminum, mercury, and lead which get in to the water which we drink. It seems that we are surrounded by aluminum. It is probable that parts of our brains get destroyed by traces of aluminum that gets in to our bodies from various sources. Kidney failures may be caused due to continuous exposure to aluminum, and could warrant use of kidney dialysis regularly. The work of removing waste from the body is taken over by kidney dialysis from the kidneys. Dialysis involves rinsing out the space between intestines and the intestinal walls with several gallons of fluid at least a couple of times a week to remove body waste which would have been carried out by urine under functioning kidneys circumstances. Aluminum gets accumulated in the bone marrow cells which are responsible for the formation of red blood cells. Consequently, these bone marrow cells are unable to utilize iron, which results in iron deficiency and the negative outcome associated with it. Aluminum can slowly accumulate in our tissues over a life time to cause thinning of bones and brain damage.

ARSENIC is another hazardous substance that is absorbed by our bodies through air pollution, antibiotics given to commercial live stocks, certain marine plants, chemical processing plants, coal fired power plants, defoliants, drinking water, fish, herbicides, insecticides, meats raised by commercially raised cattle, poultry, metal ore smelting, pesticides, oysters, mussels, wood preservatives, etc. Its overall hazardous affect is on all organs, gastrointestinal system, lungs, skin, etc. Excessive levels of arsenic can cause stomach pain, burning mouth and throat, lung and skin cancer, diarrhea, nausea, skin lesions, peripheral vascular problems, vascular collapse, etc.

CADMIUM comes in to our bodies through air pollution, art supplies, bone meal, cigarette smoke, coffee, fruit, grains, vegetables grown in cadmium laden soil, highway dust, fungicides, fresh water fish, animal kidneys and livers, refined foods, poultry, incinerators, nickel cadmium batteries, mining, fumes from welding, tobacco and its smoke, sewage sludge, smelting plants, softened water, power plants, phosphate fertilizers, paints, oxide dusts, crabs, flounder, scallops, mussels, oysters, etc. It adversely affects the brain in general, pain centers in brain, heart and blood vessels, kidneys and lungs, appetite, etc. Arsenic causes anemia, dry and scaly skin, yellow teeth, pain in the back, lung cancer, leg pain, cardio vascular disease (CVD), emphysema, fatigue, hair loss, heart disease, joint pain, hyper tension, depressed immune system response, kidney stones, liver damage, loss of appetite and sense of smell, etc. Besides, the usual healing process, the stroke patients have to be careful about their diets, and environment.

We receive **LEAD** in our bodies from air pollution, ammunition (bullets) cast iron porcelain steel bathtubs, canned foods, batteries, chemical fertilizers, ceramics, gasoline, dolomite dust, foods grown around industrial area, cosmetics, hair dyes and rinses, newsprints and color advertisements, leaded glass, paints, pesticides, pewter pottery, rubber toys, soft coal, tobacco smoke, tap water, vinyl mini blinds, etc. It adversely affects the brain, heart, bones, kidneys, pancreas, liver, nervous system, etc. Lead causes anemia, anorexia, anxiety, stomach pain, exhaustion, brain damage, bone pain, constipation, confusion, dizziness, convulsions, drowsiness, headache, brain damage, hyper tension, concentration difficulties, indigestion, loss of appetite, loss of muscle coordination, memory difficulties, miscarriage, etc. Dr. R, Casdorph and Dr. M Walker describe in book (Toxic Metal Syndrome) that 4 million tons of lead is mined each year, and existing levels in the environment are 500 times higher than pre-historic levels.

Toxicity of lead is widely known, and even a short time exposure to children and pregnant women can be dangerous to their health. Still many people believe that once the lead containing paint was banned from their homes, the dangers from lead poisoning were over. Later when the lead was banned in gasoline, people thought the danger from lead is completely over. No, it is not over. Lead is in our environment, and people of all income levels, ethnicities, and locations are being affected. This is a great burden on stroke patients who are trying to get well. Lead is a known neurotoxin which kills brain cells. Higher levels of lead in blood can cause learning disabilities. It causes attention deficit disorder, and reduced intelligence. Stroke patients are in the process of re-learning all those things they used to know.

MERCURY is a known poison. In high or pure doses it is lethal. We receive this poison through air pollution, batteries, cosmetics, dental amalgams diuretics, electrical devices, relays, explosives, fungicides, grains, fluorescent lights, large bass, pike, trout, large halibut, snappers, sword fish, shrimp, shell fish, tap water, insecticides, pesticides, paints, petroleum products, etc. Mercury affects the pain centers in brain, cell membranes, nervous system, kidneys, etc. In excessive levels, Mercury causes abnormality in nervous development, anorexia, anemia, anxiety, blindness, blue line on gums, depression, colitis, dermatitis, difficulty in chewing and swallowing, depression, dizziness, drowsiness, hyper tension, headache, emotional instability, nerve damage, memory loss, vision impairment, inflamed gums, insomnia, kidney damage, metallic taste, loss of smell, hearing loss, hallucinations, fatigue, fever, loss of appetite, loss of muscles, loss of weight, etc. Dr. Maile Pouls who suffered from mercury poisoning is a great believer in chelating therapy, and believes that it will save lives and billions of dollars.

Among the most common sources of exposure to Mercury is from silver dental fillings. About 225 million Americans have dental fillings. Fillings contain about 50% mercury when placed in teeth. Mercury fillings release microscopic particles and vapors of mercury each and every time a person chews. Particles get absorbed and vapors are inhaled. Mercury particles absorption takes place in tooth roots, mucous membranes, of the mouth and gums, and in the stomach lining. Mercury levels range between 20 and 400 mcg/m3 in the mouth and there remains a continuous exposure. Various researches have been conducted on the affects of mercury in the dental fillings and various fish with varied outcomes. Dr. Mark Hulet's research outcomes on Amalgam fillings are: the experience of depression, suicidal impulses, irritability, inability to cope, muscle spasms, seizures, multiple sclerosis, cardio vascular problems, accelerated heart beat, facial tics, arthritis, bursitis, immune system diseases, airborne allergies, food allergies, effects on psychological reactions, etc. According to Dr. Hal Higgins who conducted several research analysis when American Dental Association, Environmental Protection Agency, and several others were conducting several studies on the impact of mercury on Amalgam fillings, found that all researchers believed that continuous exposure to mercury results from mercury in the dental fillings. However, almost all researchers differ on the level of danger it poses to the body. Therefore, the results are contentious.

Yet there is another metal which is hazardous. It is **NICKEL**. We receive exposure to nickel from ceramics, appliances, cocoa, cooking utensils, coins, cosmetics, dental materials, hydrogenated oils, chocolate, nuts, foods grown near industrial areas, industrial waste, hair spray, medical implants, jewelry, metal refineries, nickel cadmium batteries, metal tools, orthodontic appliances, shampoos, solid waste incinerators, kitchen utensils made of stainless steel, tap water, tobacco and its smoke, water faucets and pipes, zippers, etc. Nickel affects the larynx (voice box), areas of skin exposed to it, lungs, nasal passages, etc. Nickel causes blue colored lips, vomiting, headache, rapid heart rate, shortness of breath, skin rashes, insomnia, diarrhea, fever, cancer of lung, larynx and nasal passage, gingivitis, etc. People living in and around the vicinity of nickel smelting and refining plants may be exposed to excessive amounts of nickel. I saw and heard about these symptoms in person during my several visits to Sudbury, Ontario. Obviously, it is not an easy task to get well fast when the patient has to face so many dangers from so many sources at once, besides the health danger from within. It is the accumulative burden that is so burdensome on the patient that makes it a compelling reason to be as cautious as the circumstances allow for the patients to get better, without experiencing the subsequent stroke or heart attack.

The famous names associated with metals in the environment and their health impact on humans are: Omegatech King James Medical Lab, Cleveland, OH, California Preventive Medicine Foundation, Center for Occupational & Environmental Medicine (Dr. James Scheer), Great Smokey's Diagnostic Lab (Dr. Bob Smith), Dr. Elmer Cranston (author of Passing Bypass, Dr. D. R. McLaughlin, Researcher, University of Toronto, and many others.

If you are not eating healthy, then start eating healthy. Develop a good **METABOLISM**. For the day to day function of our bodies, we need chemical energy for which we need to consume calories from the food sources. To convert food calories in to chemical energy, we require a metabolic process. A good metabolism converts food calories in to chemical energy efficiently and with minimum effort. Eating a lot does not mean a high metabolism. Inadequate diets, improper breathing and poor digestion are very common reasons for poor metabolism. Depressed state of mind can cause digestive problems, poor breathing, and lack of activities, etc. Poor breathing and lack of activities can lead to insufficient supply of oxygen in the body, which is necessary to burn the food we eat. This also causes lack of circulation, diabetes, and associated diseases. Mind can play tricks on our bodies. A depressed mind can influence the immune system, thereby, causing problems associated with our nervous system, stomach, etc. Therefore, healthy and adequate diets are essential for patients and for an ordinary person as well.

Also, avoiding exposure to toxins, chemical pollution, etc. in the environment should become an important point of life style. DNA in our bodies has all the information to trouble shoot and cure any ailment or dysfunction in the body. Toxins and pollution can damage DNA which contains the vital and crucial information for the patient to get well. Aged people have lower immune system than the younger ones and, therefore, it becomes much more important for aged to avoid toxins and pollution.

Stroke and heart attack patients should choose foods from lower chain of life. Eating of animal flesh should be minimum, if cannot be avoided completely. Avoid or minimize consuming animal protein. We should eat preferably just the right amount of total protein that our body requires to make and repair tissues. The excess amount of protein, then, will be used as energy source of fuel. Protein molecules are big and quite complicated, and their digestion requires much more work out than carbohydrates and fats. Energy output from consuming protein is less efficient as compared to that of other nutrients. According to Dr. Andrew Weil, protein fuel does not burn clean. Protein contains nitrogen, and after metabolism it leaves a toxic nitrogenous residue which eventually goes to the liver where it turns to urea which, in turn is flushed out by the kidneys. It is a burdensome task for the liver and kidneys to process this toxin, which can weaken the immune system temporarily. About 60 grams of protein per day is more than enough for an adult. Stroke and heart patients must consider looking in to this daily intake of protein, and consult the attending physician. Whereas, carbohydrates and fats are composed of carbon, hydrogen, and oxygen, and after metabolism carbon dioxide and water are left. Energy from carbohydrates and non animal fats is efficient and considerably easy to burn with no negative affects.

FOODS

Certain kind of fish is ideal source of PROTEIN. The fish as a source of protein would be that which has lower levels of AA (harmful fatty acids) than EPA (beneficial) fatty acids. Not all fish is good. There are some which are best, and should be preferred, then there are second best which should be considered, then there are fish which require EPA supplement, and then there are fish which should be avoided by stroke and heart patients. Besides, one should be careful consuming too much of fish because certain fish is believed to contain unsafe quantities of mercury.

According to CHILTON PROGRAM, developed by Dr. Floyd Chilton, the best fish are: European Anchovies, Atlantic/Pacific Herring, Atlantic/Pacific Mackerel, wild Chinook salmon, Roe, black and red caviar, wild Sockeye salmon. The second best choice is: wild pink salmon, Greenland halibut, wild Coho salmon, Alaskan king crab, blue crab, wild Chum salmon, smelt, shrimp, wild oysters, farmed oysters, mussels, sea bass, white tuna, squid.

The third best choice is: scallops, clams, flounder, rainbow trout, yellow fin tuna, trout, swordfish, walleye, sardines, wild Atlantic salmon, haddock, Atlantic cod, perch, snapper, mahi mahi, tilefish. These fish do contain sufficient beneficial fatty acids and, therefore, EPA supplement may be taken while consuming such fish. Your doctor will be able to recommend the exact amount of fish and the dosage of EPA supplement.

Then there are fish which should be avoided, because they contain high levels of AA, the harmful fatty acids: grouper, Atlantic/Pacific halibut, Florida pompano, farmed channel catfish, wild channel catfish, farmed Atlantic salmon.

Coincidently, not all the people who suffer from a stroke or heart attack are financially well off. Only a few patients will be able to afford the high priced fish which will provide a well balanced AA/EPA ratio. For those, who are unable to afford such expensive fish, they are blessed with a host of alternatives to fish. These alternatives are vegetarian foods which happen to be ideal diet after suffering from a stroke or heart attack, because they do not cause any burden to the cardio vascular system of the body. Here is some information that might be of some help to you in choosing the appropriate foods from the non-animal product source for your specific needs.

FOODS YOU SHOULD INCORPORATE IN YOUR DIET

NON ANIMAL SOURCES OF NUTRITION

*Thanks to Dr. Decuypere of Health Alternatives, and many others for the compilation of nutritional values in the following mentioned foods.

BEANS & LENTILS

BLACK BEANS (one cup cooked & drained) contains 15 grams of protein, 47 mg of calcium, 239 mg of phosphorus, 2.9 mg of iron and 609 mg of potassium

GREAT NORTHER BEANS (one cup cooked & drained): 14 grams of protein, 90 mg of calcium, 266 mg of phosphorus, 4.9 mg of iron, and 749 mg of potassium,

CHICK PEAS (one cup cooked & drained): contains 15 grams of protein, 80 mg of calcium, 273 mg of phosphorus, 4.9 mg of iron, and 475 mg of potassium.

LENTILS: (one cup cooked & drained): contains 16 grams of protein, 50 mg of calcium, 238 mg of phosphorus, 4.2 mg of iron, 498 mg of potassium, 40 IU of vitamin A

SOYBEANS (one cup cooked & drained): contains 20 grams of protein, 131 mg of calcium, 322 mg of phosphorus, 4.9 mg of iron, 972 mg of potassium, 50 IU of vitamin A

Besides very nutritious Moong Bean, Kidney Beans, Pinto Beans, there is large variety of other beans and lentils in the marketplace.

NUTS & SEEDS

ALMONDS: 1 ounce (about 24 whole almonds) contains 6 grams of protein, 3.35 grams of fiber, 8.2 mcg of foliate, 7.3 mg of vitamin E, 2.8 I.U. of vitamin A, 1.1 mg of niacin, 206 mg of potassium, 134 mg of phosphorus, 70 mg of calcium, 0.2 mg of sodium, 77 mg of magnesium, 1.2 mcg of selenium, 1.2 mg of iron, 0.95 mg of zinc, 0.7 mg of manganese,

BRAZIL NUTS: one ounce (about 7 whole nuts) contains 4 grams of protein, 2.1 grams of fiber, 6.24 mcg of foliate, 1.6 mg of vitamin E, 1.0 mg of vitamin C, 205 mg of phosphorus, 186.8 mg of potassium, 106 mg of magnesium, 543 mcg of selenium, 45 mg of calcium, 1.15 mg of zinc, and 0.69 mg of iron

CASHEW NUTS:: one ounce raw whole nuts contain 5.17 gm of protein, 0.94 gm of fiber, 9.7 mcg of vitamin K, 7.0 mcg of foliate, 187 mg of potassium, 168 mg of phosphorus, 82.8 mg of magnesium, 10.5 mg of calcium, 3.4 mg of sodium, 1.9 mg of iron, and 1.64 mg of zinc, and 5.6 mg of selenium.

CHESTNUTS: 10 roasted kernels with no salt added contain 2.7 grams of protein, 4.3 grams of fiber, 20 I.U. of vitamin A, 21.8 mg of vitamin C, 1.12 mg of niacin, 0.46 mg of pantothenic acid, 58.8 mcg of foliate, 6.55 mcg of vitamin K, 497 mg of potassium, 90 mg of phosphorus, 24.4 mg of calcium, 27.7 mg of magnesium, 1.7 mg of sodium, 0.76 mg of iron, 1.0 mcg of selenium, 1.0 mg of manganese,

HAZELNUTS: 10 raw nuts contain 2 grams of protein, 1.4 grams of fiber, 2.8 I.U. of vitamin A, 0.9 mg of vitamin C, 15.8 mcg of foliate, 2 mcg of vitamin K, 95 mg of potassium, 40.6 mg of phosphorus, 22.8 mg of magnesium, 16 mg of calcium, 0.66 mg of iron.

MACADAMIA NUTS: one ounce (about 11 kernels), raw, contains 2.24 grams of protein, 2.44 grams of fiber, 3.1 mcg of foliate, 104 mg of potassium, 53 mg of phosphorus, 36.9 mg of magnesium, 24 mg of calcium, 1.4 mg of sodium, 1.0 mg of iron.

PECANS: one ounce (about 20 halves), raw, contains 2.6 grams of protein, 2.7 grams of fiber, 15.8 I.U. of vitamin A, 6.23 mcg of foliate, 116 mg of potassium, 78 gm of phosphorus, 34.3 mg of magnesium, 19.8 mg of calcium, 1.3 mg of zinc, 0.7 mg of iron, 1.3 mg of manganese, 1.0 mcg of selenium.

PEANUTS: one ounce raw contains 7.3 grams of protein, 1.0 gm of fiber, 3.4 mg of niacin, 3.4 mg of vitamin E, 68 mcg of foliate, 200 mg of potassium, 107 mg of phosphorus, 47.6 mg of magnesium, 26 mg of calcium, 5.1 mg of sodium, 1.3 mg of iron, 2.0 mcg of selenium.

PINE NUTS: one ounce contains 3.9 grams of protein, 1.0 gram of fiber, 2.6 mg of vitamin E, 1.2 mg of niacin, 19 mcg of foliate, 8.2 I.U. of vitamin A, 15.3 mcg of vitamin K, 169 mg of potassium, 163 mg of phosphorus, 71 mg of magnesium, 4.5 mg of calcium, 2.4 mg of manganese, 1.8 mg of zinc, 1.6 mg of iron.

PISTACIO NUTS: one ounce (about 49 kernels) dry roasted contains 6.0 grams of protein, 3.0 grams of fiber, 74.3 I.U. of vitamin A, 14.2 mcg of foliate, 295.4 mg of potassium, 137 mg of phosphorus, 34 mg of magnesium, 31.2 mg of calcium, 2.8 mg of sodium, 1.2 mg of iron, 2.6 mcg of selenium.

PUMPKIN SEEDS: one ounce roasted without salt contains 5.3 mg of protein, no fiber, 17.6 I.U. of vitamin A, 2.6 mcg of foliate, 260 mg of potassium, 74 gm of magnesium, 26 mg of phosphorus, 15.6 mg of calcium, 5.1 mg of sodium, 2.9 mg of zinc, 0.9 mg of iron.

SUNFLOWER SEEDS: one ounce, dry roasted, contains 5.5 mg of protein, 3.1 mg of fiber, 6.5 I.U. of vitamin A, 67.2 mcg of foliate, 6.0 mg of vitamin E, 327.2 mg of phosphorus, 241 mg of potassium, 36.6 mg of magnesium, 19.8 mg of calcium, 1.5 mg of zinc, 0.9 mg of iron.

WALNUTS: one ounce, (about 14 halves) contains 4.3 mg of protein, 1.9 mg of fiber, 27.8 mcg of foliate, 125 mg of potassium, 98.0 mg of phosphorus, 44.8 mg of magnesium, 27.8 mg of calcium, 1.0 mg of zinc, 0.8 mg of iron, 1.4 mcg of selenium.

FRUITS

APPLE: one medium apple with skin contains no protein, 4 grams of fiber, 73 I.U. of vitamin A, 9 mg of vitamin C, 4 mcg of foliate, 0.66 I.U. of vitamin E, 158 mg of potassium, 9.5 mg of calcium, 9.5 mg of phosphorus, 7 mg of magnesium, and 4 mg of selenium.

AVOCADO: one medium, contains 4 gm of protein, 10 gm of fiber, 1230 I.U. of vitamin A, 15.9 mg of vitamin C, 3.9 mg of niacin, 124 mcg of foliate, 1.9 mg of pentothenic acid, 0.56 mg of vitamin B6, 0.2 mg of vitamin B1, 0.25 mg of vitamin B2, 1204 mg of potassium, 82.4 mg of phosphorus, 78.4 mg of magnesium, 22 mg of calcium, 20 mg of sodium, 2 mg of iron.

BANANA: one medium, contains 1 gram of protein, 3 grams of fiber, 95 I.U. of vitamin A, 11 mg of vitamin C, 22.5 mcg of foliate, 0.7 mg of vitamin B6, 0.6 mg of niacin, 0.31 mcg of pentothenic acid, 0.67 mg of vitamin E, 467 mg of potassium, 43 mg of magnesium, 27 mg of phosphorus, 7 mg of calcium, 1.3 mg of selenium, 0.4 mg of iron.

BLACKBERRIES: one cup contains 1 gram of protein, 7 grams of fiber, 237 I.U. of vitamin A, 30 mg of vitamin C, 1.5 mg of vitamin E, 49 mcg of foliate, 282 mg of potassium, 46 mg of calcium, 30 mg of phosphorus, 28 mg of magnesium, 1.9 mg of manganese, 0.8 mg of iron, 0.9 mg of selenium, 0.4 mg of zinc.

CANTALOUPE: one medium slice contains 0.6 grams of protein, 0.55 grams of fiber, 2225 I.U. of vitamin A, 3.7 mg of vitamin C, 3.9 mg of foliate, 0.4 mg of niacin, 213 mg of potassium, 12 mg of phosphorus, 7.6 mg of calcium, 7.6 mg of magnesium.

GRAPES; one cup contains one gram of protein, 1.6 grams of fiber, 92 I.U. of vitamin A, 3.7 mg of vitamin C, 3.6 mcg of foliate, 176 mg of potassium, 13 mg of calcium, 9 mg of phosphorus, 4.6 mg of magnesium, 0.4 mg of iron, 0.3 mg of selenium.

KIWI: one cup contains 1.75 grams of protein, 6 grams of fiber, 310 I.U. of vitamin A, 174 mg of vitamin C, 67 mcg of foliate, 3 I.U of vitamin E, less than 1 mg of vitamins B2 and B6, 0.9 mg of niacin, 588 mg of potassium, 71 mg of phosphorus, 53 mg of magnesium, 46 mg of calcium, 1.1 mg of selenium, 0.72 mg of iron, 0.3 mg of zinc, 0.3 mg of copper.

LEMON: one without peel contains .64 grams of protein, 1.6 grams of fiber, 2 I.U. of vitamin A, 4 mg of vitamin C, 80 mg of potassium, 15 mg of calcium, 9.2 mg of phosphorus, 4.6 mg of magnesium, 0.35 mg of iron,.

LIME: one, without peel, contains 0.4 grams of protein, 1.8 grams of fiber, 6.7 I.U of vitamin A, 19 mg of vitamin C, 5.5 mcg of foliate, 68 mg of potassium, 22 mg of calcium, 12 mg of phosphorus, 4 mg of magnesium, 0.4 mg of iron.

MANGO; one without the peel, contains 1 gram of protein, 3 grams of fiber, 8060 I.U. of vitamin A, 57 mg of vitamin C, 29 mcg of foliate, 1.2 mg of niacin, 3.51 I.U of vitamin E, less than 1 mg each of vitamins B2 and B6, 323 mg of potassium, 20.7 mg of calcium, 22.8 mg of phosphorus, 18.6 mg of magnesium, 0.26 mg of iron.

ORANGE: one medium, contains 1 gram of protein, 3 grams of fiber, 269 I.U. of vitamin A, 70 mg of vitamin C, 40 mcg of foliate, less than 1 mg each of vitamin B1 and pantothenic acid, 237 mg of potassium, 52 mg of calcium, 18 mg of magnesium, 0.65 mg of selenium.

PEACH: one medium with skin, contains no protein, 1 gram of fiber, 524 I.U of vitamin A, 19 mg of vitamin C, 5.5 mcg of foliate, 0.97 mg of niacin, 193 mg of potassium, 12 mg of phosphorus, 6.9 mg of magnesium, 5 mg of calcium, 0.4 mg of selenium.

STRAWBERRIES: one cup of whole strawberries contains no protein, 3 grams of fiber, 39 I.U. of vitamin A, 82 mg of vitamin C, 25.5 mcg of foliate, 239 mg of potassium, 27 mg of phosphorus, 20 mg of calcium, 14 mg of magnesium, 1 mg of selenium, 0.55 mg of iron, 0.42 mg of manganese,

TOMATO: one medium, contains 1.05 grams of protein, 1.35 grams of fiber, 2364 I.U of vitamin A, 25 mg of vitamin C, 46 mcg of foliate, 0.94 mg of niacin, 0.1 mg of vitamin B6, 396.7 mg of potassium, 62.7 mg of phosphorus, 22.8 mg of magnesium, 31.9 mg of calcium, 11.4 mg of sodium, 0.51 mg of iron, 0.8 mg of selenium.

WATERMELON: one medium slice contains 1 gram of protein, 1 gram of fiber, 1050 I.U. of vitamin A, 27 mg of vitamin C, 0.57 mg of niacin, 6.33 mcg of foliate, 0.23 mg of vitamin B1, 0.4 mg of vitamin B6, 332 mg of potassium, 31.5 mg of magnesium, 26 mg of phosphorus, 23 mg of calcium, 0.5 mg of iron, 0.3 mg of selenium.

VEGETABLES:
ARTICHOKE: one medium cooked with no added salt, contains 4.2 grams of protein, 5.5 grams of fiber, 425 mg of potassium, 103 mg of phosphorus, 72 mg of magnesium, 54 mg of calcium, and trace amounts of selenium, iron, manganese, copper and zinc.

ASPARAGUS; ½ cup (about 4 spears) cooked with no salt added, contains 2 grams of protein, 1.5 grams of fiber, 144 mg of potassium, 48.5 mg of phosphorus, 18 mg of calcium, 10 mg of sodium, 9 mg of magnesium,

BROCCOLI: ½ cup cooked with no added salt, contains2.3 grams of protein, 2.3 grams of fiber, 228 mg of potassium, 46 mg of phosphorus, 36 mg of calcium, 28 mg of sodium, 18.7 mg of magnesium, 0.65 mg of iron,

110 mcg of vitamin K, and trace amounts of selenium, manganese, copper and zinc.

CARROTS: ½ cup cooked with no salt added, contains 0.85 grams of protein, 2.6 grams of fiber, 177 mg of potassium, 51.5 mg of sodium, 24 mg of calcium, 23.4 mg of phosphorus, 10 mg of magnesium, 0.48 mg of iron, trace amounts of selenium, manganese, copper, and zinc.

CAULIFLOWER; ½ cup cooked with no salt added, contains 1.1 grams of protein, 1.7 grams of fiber, 88 mg of potassium, 19.8 mg of phosphorus, 9.9 mg of calcium, 9.3 mg of sodium, 5.6 mg of magnesium, trace amounts of selenium, copper, iron, manganese, and zinc.

CORN: one ear cooked with no salt added, contains 2.6 grams of protein, 2.1 grams of fiber, 191.7 mg of potassium, 79 mg of phosphorus, 24.6 mg of magnesium, 13 mg of sodium, 1.5 mg of calcium, 0.6 mg of selenium, 0.5 mg of iron, 0.4 mg of zinc.

CUCUMBER: ½ a cup with skin sliced, contains 0.36 grams of protein, 0.42 grams of fiber, 74,9 mg of potassium, 1.4 mg of phosphorus, 5.7 mg of magnesium, 1 mg of sodium, 7.3 mg of calcium, trace amounts of selenium, copper, iron, manganese, and zinc.

GREEN PEPPER: 1 small raw contains 0.66 grams of protein, 1.3 grams of fiber, 14 mg of potassium, 7.4 mg of magnesium, 6.7 mg of calcium, 1.48 mg of sodium.

KALE: 1 cup of cooked with no salt added, contains 2.5 grams of protein, 2.6 grams of fiber, 296 mg of potassium, 36 mg of phosphorus, 23 mg of magnesium, 32 mg of calcium, 29.9 mg of sodium, 1.2 mg of iron, 0.5 mg of manganese, 1.2 mg of selenium, 1062 mcg of vitamin K.

LIMA BEANS: 1 cup of cooked large lima beans with no salt added, contains 14.7 grams of protein, 13.2 grams of fiber, 965 mg of potassium,

208.7 mg of phosphorus, 8.8 mg of magnesium, 32 mg of calcium, 8.5 mg of selenium, 4.5 mg of iron, 3.8 mg of sodium, 1.8 mg of zinc, 0.8 mg of manganese, 0.44 mg of copper.

MUSHROOMS: ½ cup of raw contains 1 gram of protein, 0.42 grams of fiber, 129.5 mg of potassium, 36.4 mg of phosphorus, 3.5 mg of magnesium, 3 mg of selenium, 1.8 mg of calcium, 1.4 mg of sodium, 0.36 mg of iron.

ONIONS: 1 small cooked without salt added, contains 0.8 grams of protein, 1.3 grams of fiber, 110 mg of potassium, 23 mg of phosphorus, 14 mg of calcium, 7 mg of magnesium, 2.1 mg of sodium, 0.42 mg of selenium.

PEAS: 1 cup boiled with no salt added contains 8.58 grams of protein, 8.8 grams of fiber, 433.6 mg of potassium, 187 mg of phosphorus, 62 mg of magnesium, 43 mg of calcium, 4.8 mg of sodium, 2.5 mg of iron, 3 mg of selenium, 1.9 mg of zinc, 0.8 mg of manganese.

POTATOES: 1 medium baked with no salt added, contains 3 grams of protein, 2.3 grams of fiber, 610 mg of potassium, 78 mg of phosphorus, 39 mg of magnesium, 7.8 mg of calcium, 7.8 mg of sodium, 0.55 mg of iron, 0.46 mg of selenium, 0.45 mg of zinc.

SPINACH: one cup of uncooked contains 0.86 grams of protein, 0.81 grams of fiber, 167 mg of potassium, 14.7 mg of phosphorus, 23.7 mg of magnesium, 29.7 mg of calcium, 23.7 mg of sodium, 145 mcg of vitamin K.

SQUASH, SUMMER, ZUCCHINI, one cup of sliced without salt, contains 1.65 grams of protein, 2.5 grams of fiber, 345.6 mg of potassium, 7 mg of phosphorus, 43 mg of magnesium, 48.6 mg of calcium, 1.8 mg of sodium, 0.65 mg of iron, 0.38 mg of manganese, 0.36 mg of selenium, 0.7 mg of zinc.

SQUASH, WINTER: one cup of cubed, baked with no salt added, contains 1.02 grams of protein, 2.07 grams of fiber, 181 mg of potassium, 21.7 mg of phosphorus, 17 mg of magnesium, 32.5 mg of calcium, 27.9 mg of sodium, 0.52 mg of iron, 0.46 mg of selenium,

SWEET POTATOES: one medium, baked in its own skin, contains 1.96 grams of protein, 3.42 grams of fiber, 273 mg of potassium, 29.5 mg of phosphorus, 13.5 mg of magnesium, 6.2 mg of calcium, 11 mg of sodium, 0.55 mg of iron, 0.5 mg of selenium, .06 mg of manganese, 0.3 mg of zinc.

The nutritional values are just approximate just to acquaint the patients and non-patients to the over all values of the most common foods that are consumed. Knowledge of such nutritional values help us to diversify our meal menus for the optimal intake of right amounts of various foods in conjunction with the supplements we take on a daily basis, either voluntarily or through prescriptions. In the following line, a brief description of the known benefits that are available to our bodies by consuming each specific vitamin through our daily food, as well as, through supplements.

RECOMMENDED NUTRITION INTAKE & ITS SOURCES

VITAMIN A
10,000 I.U. (plant derived) per day are recommended for adult males, and 8,000 I.U. for adult females (12,000 I.U. if lactating). Vitamin A helps in cell reproduction, it stimulates immune system, and is required for the formation of some hormones. It helps our vision, bone growth, development of teeth, healthy skin, hair, and mucous membranes. It has been identified to affect prevention against measles. Vitamin A deficiency can cause night blindness, dry skin, poor bone growth, and poor tooth enamel. Beta Carotene, alpha carotene and retinol are versions of vitamin A. A significant amount of vitamin A can be sourced from cantaloupes, tomatoes, oranges, kiwi, peaches, water-

melon, blackberries, sweet potatoes, kale, green peppers, summer squash (zuc-chini), carrots, spinach, avocado, asparagus, peas, and broccoli.

VITAMIN B-1 (thiamine):

1.2 mg for adult males and 1.1 mg for females (1.5 mg if lactating) are rec-ommended for consumption each day. Vitamin B-1 (thiamine) helps the body to convert carbohydrates in our food to energy. Therefore, it is important for the production of energy in our body. It is essential for func-tioning of the heart muscles, and the nervous system. Most fruits and veg-etables are not sufficient in thiamin. Its deficiency can cause fatigue and general weakness in our body. It is available in varied quantities in peas, avocado, and watermelon.

VITAMIN B-2 (riboflavin):

1.3 mg for adult males and 1.1 mg for females (1.5 mg if pregnant or lactating) are recommended for consumption each day. Vitamin B-2 is important for the body growth, and the reproduction of red cells. It helps in releasing energy from the carbohydrates. Most fruits and vegetables are not a significant source of this vitamin. Kiwi and avocado contain some quantities of this vitamin.

VITAMIN B-3 (niacin):

16 mg for adult males and 14 mg for women (17 to 18 mg if pregnant or lactating) are recommended for consumption each day. Vitamin B-3 is important for conversion of food to energy. It assists in the functioning digestive system and nerves. It also aids the health of skin. Prominent sources of this vitamin are corn, artichoke, asparagus, summer squash (zucchini), lima beans, sweet potatoes, kale, broccoli, carrots, green pep-pers, peanuts, pine nuts, chestnuts, almonds.

VITAMIN B-5 (pantothenic acid)

5 mg for adult men and women (6 to 7 mg for women who are pregnant or lactating) are recommended for consumption on daily basis. It is essen-tial for the metabolism of food in the body. Also, it is essential for the pro-duction of hormones, and the good cholesterol. Oranges, bananas,

avocado, sweet potatoes, potatoes, corn, lima beans, winter squash, artichokes, mushrooms, broccoli, cauliflower, carrots, are good sources of this vitamin.

VITAMIN B-6 (pyridoxine)
1.3 mg to 1.7 mg for male and female adults (2 mg for women who are pregnant or lactating) are recommended for daily consumption. Vitamin B-6 is required for the chemical reaction of proteins. Higher the protein is consumed, then higher the need for vitamin B-6 becomes. It plays an important role in the creation of antibodies in the immune system, and also acts in the formation of red blood cells. Besides, it helps to maintain normal nerve function. Shortage of vitamin B-6 in the diet can cause convulsions, irritability, confusion, dizziness, and nausea. Good sources of this vitamin are watermelon, bananas, avocado, peas, potatoes, carrots.

VITAMIN B-7 (biotin)
30 mcg to 100 mcg for adult males and females, and pregnant/lactating women are recommended. Along with other vitamin B s, biotin helps convert food in to energy. For healthy hair, skin, and nails it is especially important. Good sources of biotin are soy beans, broccoli, sweet potatoes, sunflower seeds, and some nuts. Signs of biotin deficiency are hair loss, nausea, vomiting, muscle pain, fatigue, red inflamed tongue, loss of appetite, skin rashes.

VITAMIN B-9 (foliate/folic acid)
400 mcg for male and female adults (500 mcg to 600 mcg for pregnant/lactating women) are recommended for daily consumption. Healthy nails, hair, skin, mucous membranes, nerves, and blood depend on vitamin B-9. Foliate/folic acid is essential for the production of red blood cells, as well as, components of nervous system. Also, it helps in the creation and formation process of RNA and DNA. It is a critical part of spinal fluid. It is important for the maintenance of brain function. It is absolutely essential for proper cell growth and the development of embryo. Women who are pregnant are recommended to take foliate/folic acid in sufficient quantities

on daily basis. Prominent sources of this vitamin are: kiwi, blackberries, tomatoes, oranges, strawberries, bananas, cantaloupe, lima beans, asparagus, avocado, peas, artichoke, spinach, winter squash, broccoli, summer squash (zucchini), corn, sweet potatoes, kale, potatoes, carrots, onions, green peppers, peanuts, sunflower seeds, chestnuts, walnuts, hazelnuts, pine nuts.

VITAMIN B-12
2.4 mcg for male and female adults and 2.6 to 2.8 mcg for pregnant and lactating women are recommended for daily consumption. Like other B vitamins, it is important for our metabolism. Vitamin B-12 helps in the formation of red blood cells, and in the maintenance of central nervous system of the body. The only known sources of this vitamin are fish, meat, poultry, and dairy products.

VITAMIN C
60 mg for male and female adults, 70 mg for pregnant women, and 95 mg for those who are lactating are recommended for daily consumption. This is among the important vitamins in providing protection to the body. It plays a significant role as an antioxidant, and protects the body tissue from the damage of oxidation. Body's metabolism's byproduct free radicals are potentially damaging. Free radicals can cause cell damage which, in turn, contributes to cardio vascular disease (CVD) and cancer. As an antioxidant, vitamin C protects the body from these free radicals. Vitamin C is also an affective anti-viral agent. Prominent sources of this vitamin are: tomatoes, lime, peach, bananas, apples, lemon, grapes, cucumber, green peppers, kale, lima beans, mushrooms, onions, peas, potatoes, spinach, summer squash (zucchini), winter squash, and sweet potatoes.

VITAMIN D
5 mg for male and female adults, 10 mg for male and female adults between 50 years and 70 years, and 15 mg for adults above 70 years. Our bodies manufacture this vitamin after being exposed to sun for about 15 minutes. Vitamin D is vital to the body, and without this calcium and

magnesium do not get absorbed by the body. Calcium and phosphorus are essential for the development of healthy bones and teeth, and therefore vitamin D becomes crucial to their proper absorption and maintenance of balance. Recent research shows that vitamin D is a lot more important than its current known role of aiding absorption of calcium and magnesium. Vitamin D deficiency has been linked to a lot of ailments and cancer. Therefore, it is advisable to take adequate dosages of this vitamin, especially if you are a stroke or heart patient.

VITAMIN E
30 I.U. of male and female adults is recommended for daily consumption. Just like vitamin C, this vitamin also acts like an antioxidant to protect body tissues from the damage caused by oxidation. It prevents free radicals from damaging cells and tissues. In this way, vitamin E deters atherosclerosis and accelerates wound healing. It helps to minimize the wrinkles, heals minor wounds, and soothes the broken or stressed skin tissue. It plays an important role in the formation of red blood cells and the absorption of vitamin K. Prominent sources of this vitamin are: blackberries, bananas, apples, almonds, sunflower seeds, pine nuts, peanuts, Brazil nuts.

VITAMIN K
70 mcg to 80 mcg for male adults, and 60 mcg to 65 mcg for female adults are recommended for daily consumption. This vitamin is naturally produced by the bacteria in our intestines. It is needed to form essential proteins, for blood clotting, kidney function, and bone metabolism. Prominent sources of this vitamin are: spinach, turnip greens, broccoli, cabbage, kale, and other leafy vegetables, pine nuts, cashew nuts, chestnuts, hazelnuts.

PROTEIN is an essential nutrient for the body. Protein is required to make new tissue, to grow it, maintain it, and repair it as when it is required. Protein is made of a variety of Amino Acids. Some of these amino acids cannot be made by our bodies and, therefore, must be received through our diet. Protein deficiency causes retarded growth, and also the lack of sufficient protein results in slow healing ability. Meat, poultry, fish, and dairy products are the non vegetarian sources of protein. Beans, lentils grains, nuts, and seeds are the vegetarian sources of protein in our diet. Please note that most vegetables contain some protein, even though the quantity is insignificant. Protein from animal source is concentrated, while the protein from agricultural source is less concentrated.

MINERALS
CALCIUM
1000 mg for male and female adults are recommended for daily consumption. Calcium helps in the absorption of nutrients through the cell walls. It helps us to sleep, and tend to ease up the insomnia condition. Calcium deficiency can cause difficulties in the contraction of muscles, failure of nerves to carry messages, and clotting of blood, muscle spasms, cramps, etc. Under calcium deficient conditions, the body takes calcium from the bones, which makes the bones weaker and brittle. Brittle bones can break easily. For stroke patients and seniors, it becomes very important to maintain adequate levels of calcium in the food intake, as this is the time when osteoporosis sets in if the body is denied of calcium. Prominent sources of calcium are: orange, blackberries, kiwi, tomatoes, lime, strawberries, lemon, grapes, apples, cantaloupe, bananas, peach, artichoke, peas, summer squash, broccoli, kale, lima beans, winter squash, spinach, carrots, avocado, asparagus, almonds, Brazil nuts, pistachio nuts, walnuts, chestnuts, macadamia nuts, pecans, sunflower seeds, hazelnuts, cashews, pumpkin seeds, pine nuts.

COPPER
1.3 mg to 3 mg per day for male and female adults is recommended. Copper helps in the absorption, metabolism, and storage of iron in our bodies. It also helps in the supply of oxygen to the body, as well as in the formation process of red blood cells. Copper deficiency will cause lack of iron, and will result in anemia. Prominent sources of iron are: apples, bananas, blackberries, cantaloupe, grapes, kiwi lemon, lime, orange, peach, strawberry, tomatoes, lima beans, artichoke, avocado, broccoli, carrots, cauli-

flower, corn, cucumber, green peppers, kale, mushrooms, onions, peas, potatoes, spinach, summer and winter squash, sweet potatoes.

IODINE

150 mcg per day for male and female adults, 175 mcg per day for pregnant women are recommended. Iodine promotes healthy hair, skin, nails, and teeth. For centuries, it has been known to prevent goiter, as a part of several thyroid hormones, it strongly influences nutrient metabolism, nerve and muscle function. Its deficiency in the body may cause weight gain, hair loss, insomnia, and some forms of mental retardation. Prominent sources of this mineral are: kelp, and vegetables and nuts grown in iodine rich soil.

IRON

15 mg for adult females, 10 mg for adult males, and 30 mg for pregnant women are recommended for daily consumption. There are two kinds of dietary iron. Heme iron is found in animal products and non-heme iron which is found in dark green vegetables, grains, nuts, and dried fruits. Non-heme iron, derived from non animal source is best absorbed when consumed with vitamin C. Nuts, fruits and vegetables containing iron should be consumed simultaneously with vitamin C to obtain the best results. An important aspect to note is that vitamin E should be taken separately with an interval because if taken with iron, its affects will be neutralized. If you are a complete vegetarian, then you may require an extra dose of iron in natural form or in supplement form. Prominent sources of iron are: blackberries, kiwi, strawberries, tomatoes, bananas, grapes, lima beans, peas, avocado, kale, spinach, broccoli, summer squash, potatoes, sweet potatoes, winter squash, corn, carrots, mushrooms, and a small amount of iron in most nuts.

MAGNESIUM

320 mg to 420 mg per day for adult females and males are recommended. It is an important ingredient of bone. It is essential for healthy bones, teeth, and reduces the risk of developing osteoporosis. Adequate levels of magnesium in the

blood stream protect the body from cardio vascular disease (CVD) and stroke. Our body needs for magnesium increases with the incidence of stress and illness. As a supplement, under medical advice, it can successfully treat insomnia, muscle cramps, premenstrual syndrome, high blood pressure, angina, leg cramps due to poor blood circulation, cardio vascular disease (CVD) heart disease, stroke, and increase the chances for survival among stroke and heart attack patients. It is needed for making new cells, activating B vitamins, relaxing nerves and muscles, energy production, and in clotting blood. It also helps in the absorption of calcium, potassium, and vitamin C. Magnesium deficiency could cause fatigue, muscle weakness, heart problem, high blood pressure, insomnia, osteoporosis, and nervousness. Prominent sources of Magnesium are: kiwi, bananas, tomatoes, blackberries, strawberries, oranges, avocado, artichoke, peas, summer squash, potatoes, corn, spinach, kale, broccoli, winter squash, sweet potatoes, Brazil nuts, cashews, almonds, pumpkin seeds, pine nuts, peanuts, walnuts, macadamia nuts, pecans, sunflower seeds, pistachios, chestnuts, hazelnuts.

MANGANESE
2 to 5 mg per day for male and female adults is recommended. It is essential for proper formation and maintenance of bones, cartilages, and connective tissues. It acts as an antioxidant, and assists in normal blood clotting. It functions in enzyme reactions, thyroid hormone function, blood sugar, and metabolism. Most prominent sources of manganese are: blackberries, strawberries, peas, lima beans, sweet potatoes, kale, summer squash, pine nuts, pecans, walnuts, chestnuts.

PHOSPHORUS
800 mg per day for male and female adults (1200 mg for pregnant women) are recommended. Like calcium, it is necessary for the formation of bones, nerve cells, and teeth. Phosphorus deficiency, though rare, cause loss of appetite, general weakness, and bone pain. Prominent sources of this mineral are: kiwi, tomatoes, blackberries, bananas, strawberries, orange, peach, lime, cantaloupe, lima beans, peas, artichoke, avocado, corn, potatoes, asparagus, broccoli, kale, mushrooms, sweet potatoes, sun-

flower seeds, brazil nuts, cashews, pine nuts, pistachios, almond, peanuts, walnuts, chestnuts, pecans, macadamia nuts, hazelnuts, pumpkin seeds.

POTASSIUM

2000 mg per day for adult females and males is recommended. It is essential to maintain fluid balance, growth, and regulation of heart beat and blood pressure. It is also required for carbohydrate metabolism, insulin secretion by the pancreas, and protein synthesis. Studies suggest that people who regularly consume potassium rich foods are less likely to develop atherosclerosis, high blood pressure, heart disease, or to die of a stroke. Deficiency may cause muscle cramps, high blood pressure, heart disease, stroke, irregular heart beat, insomnia and kidney and lung failure. Prominent sources of potassium are: bananas, tomatoes, blackberries, strawberry, orange, cantaloupe, peach, grapes, apples, lemon, lime, avocado, lima beans, potatoes, peas, artichokes, summer squash, kale, sweet potatoes, broccoli, corn, winter squash, spinach, asparagus, green peppers, mushrooms, onions, cauliflower, cucumber, chestnuts, sunflower seeds, pistachios, almonds, brazil nuts, peanuts, cashews, pine nuts, walnuts, pecans, macadamia nuts, hazelnuts.

SELENIUM

70 mcg per day for male adults, 55 mcg for female adults, and 65 mcg for pregnant women are recommended. It is an antioxidant which protects cells and tissues from damage by free radicals. It supports immune system, and works in conjunction with vitamin E. Adequate levels of selenium may prevent stroke, heart disease, arthritis, and cancer. Its prominent sources are: bananas, kiwi, strawberries, blackberries, tomatoes, orange, peach, apples, grape, lima beans, peas, mushroom, kale, corn, sweet potatoes, winter squash, onions, summer squash, spinach, Brazil nuts, sunflower seeds, cashews, pistachios, peanuts, walnuts, almonds, chestnuts, pecans.

SODIUM

500 mg per day for female and male adults is recommended. All body fluids, including blood, tears, perspiration, etc. contain sodium. It regulates the blood volume and pressure, and maintains optimal pH levels. High sodium levels in the body deplete potassium, and cause the body to retain water, which causes the blood pressure to rise. A low sodium diet can reduce the high blood pressure and correct the potassium deficiency. However, overexertion can cause temporary sodium deficiency, and present symptoms of nausea, dehydration, muscle cramps, and other symptoms of stroke or heart attack. Sodium occurs in almost all fruits, vegetables, and nuts. Peanuts, pumpkin seeds, cashews, pistachios, chestnuts, macadamia nuts, and almonds do contain significant amounts.

ZINC

15 mg daily for male and female adults, 30 mg per day for pregnant women are recommended. It is integral to synthesis of RNA and DNA, the genetic material that controls cell growth, cell division, and cell function. It contributes to many body processes like: metabolism, wound healing, liver's ability to remove toxic substances, immune system, regulates the heart rate and blood pressure, Adequate zinc levels promote healthy skin and hair, short term memory and attention span. Deficiency of zinc can cause stunted growth; poor wound healing, white spots on the nails, hair loss, and fatigue. On the other hand, too much of zinc in the body can impair the immune system and produce symptoms like vomiting, fatigue, kidney problems, stomach ache. Once again, balance is the key.

HEALTHY HERBS

For clean arteries and adequate blood circulation, certain practices can be of immense help to our maintaining a healthy body. If onions, garlic, ginger, cayenne peppers, paprika, lime, whole grains, beans, lentils, olive oil, fat free milk, hard tofu, a variety of vegetables and fruits covering all ranges of color, oat bran and wheat bran, green or processed tea, and maintaining a healthy life style under non toxic environment are not a part of your current daily life, then make every effort to incorporate them in anything and everything you eat and do.

For example, unless you happen to like the taste of GARLIC, and are used to its regular use in your meals, you will find it a bit strong. Consumption of raw garlic leaves a garlic odor in mouth for several hours. Just live with it, or alternatively, let the garlic cook along with the food, in which case the garlic will not have any residual odor. Garlic is member of onion family of plants, and it has been a part of daily food of peoples around the world for thousands of years. Also, it has been considered a medicinal plant in many cultures who considered it to possess healing properties. Garlic has sulfur containing compounds with biological activity, with numerous benefits. Some of the most beneficial effects of garlic are on Cardio Vascular System. Its regular consumption can lower the blood pressure tremendously. Additionally, it lowers the blood cholesterol and blood fats (triglycerides). It increases the supply of the good cholesterol (HDL). It also stops the bad cholesterol (LDL) to get oxidized. LDL oxidization causes damage to the arterial walls. Garlic offers a noticeable protection against the cardio vascular disease (CVD). Garlic is also an antiseptic and an antibiotic which discourage the growth of many kinds of bacteria and fungi in the body. It enhances the immune system by increasing the number of killer cells that check the spread of many diseases. It contains antioxidant compounds which makes garlic to protect liver and the brain cells from degenerative changes. It also lowers blood sugar. What a great addition to the daily meal for stroke and heart patients and also for non patients. Garlic is used in almost every dish prepared in India, China, and the Far Eastern countries, also in Mediterranean and Eastern European countries

There is another very important food item and that is GINGER which has been popular as a food as well as a medicine for thousands of years in older cultures, especially in India, China, and other eastern countries where it is used almost in every meal. When consumed, it provides a warming effect and helps the digestion. It settles upset stomach, and relieves pain. It contains antioxidants and enzymes, and produces a boosting effect that boosts digestion of proteins, and protects against intestinal parasites and motion sickness. It is known to improve the blood circulation, and provides protection against cancer causing agents that can mutate the DNA.

There are a variety of HERBS that can prove to be beneficial to stroke and heart patients while recuperating from a stroke or heart attack experience, however, their use or consumption should be practiced only after a thorough study and with the guidance of a knowledgeable and sincere medical professional. In spite of all the good guidance, the patients are suggested to use these herbs in less than recommended quantities, just to see if they are workable and beneficial. All herbs have a long list of nutritional values which can be of real benefit to all people, however, they should be consumed in small quantities, so that not to allow too much nutrition of one kind to suffocate the digestive system.

To heal from a stroke or heart condition, or to avoid having one, the most prominent areas to consider will be to cut down all the deep fried foods in your diet, which can be avoided and the exercise is manageable. It is difficult to cut down all the fatty foods that we have been accustomed to eating all our lives. However, occasional consumption of favorite foods, in small portions only, prepared with caution and care for the patient, may be consumed. After all, the patient wants something good once in a while, and denying it would not serve any purpose, it will only bring aggravation to the scene. Of course, the patient would not want to forget that he/she is responsible for getting better, and he/she is in charge. Saturated fat intake should be minimized, if not completely eliminating them. Butter, margarine, whole milk, meat, poultry with skin, etc. are loaded with saturated fat and cholesterols and increased consumption of these foods can cause severe health problems. Minimize polyunsaturated vegetable oils from your diet. Develop a taste and habit of using olive oil in the preparation of your meals. Always read labels, and read the nutritional chart on the product label. Avoid the dangers of consuming Trans fatty acids (AA) which are plentiful in vegetable shortening and margarine and in the products made with partially hydrogenated oils. Develop taste for foods that contain Omega-3 fatty acids, and increase their consumption frequency. Omega-3 fatty acids are sufficiently found in fish, flax seed oil, and flaxseed meal. Just watch the adequate ratio of omega-6 and omega-3 fatty acids when consuming a certain kind of fish as mentioned in previous pages.

Eat wheat bran which contains fiber that cleans the intestinal walls, oat bran which carries out the cholesterol from the blood stream. Oat bran contains fiber which is water soluble and removes the cholesterol from the blood, which in turn, lowers the blood pressure. This is one good way to avoid having a stroke or a heart attack.

CHAPTER VII

TAKE CONTROL &
OVERCOME
DIFFICULTIES

People feel proud realizing that they are on the top of food chain on this planet. According to thousands of years old vegetarian lifestyle in India and its growing acceptance in the United States as demonstrated by Dr. Deepak Chopra, Dr. Andrew Weil, and many others, we should avoid being on top of the food chain. It is recommended that we should start eating foods on the lower chain of life. Foods that are on higher chain of life not only contain high quantities of total fat, and saturated fats, but also contain various chemicals, herbicides, pesticides, heavy metals, and other toxins which are extremely dangerous to humans. If possible, avoid animal products completely, or consume them marginally. Also, residual toxic chemicals (pesticides, herbicides, heavy metals, and fertilizing chemicals) cannot be removed from the fruits and vegetable, and therefore it is advisable to wash them thoroughly before eating them. I remember being poisoned by a 30 minute exposure to a seed dressing chemical powder. 450 workers and myself were exposed to vapors of seed dressing chemical powder (a mild herbicide) I was there just for 30 minutes and then returned to my office. Within a few days time all of my body was covered with small red spots. On checking I found all the workers had the same skin spots. A lot of vomiting, sinus problems, fever, etc. was experienced by all. We had to burn almost all the non metal accessories. Luckily no one died of the poisoning incident. Plants are grown with these seeds which are dressed with poison, and subsequent applications of pesticides and herbicides are subjected to these plants at various stages of maturity. Residues of these agricultural chemicals remain in the soil, and slowly seep in to the subsoil water table from where it gets in to our drinking water. Streams, rivers, and oceans receive quite a bit of these chemicals, which results in toxins in sea food. Therefore, organically grown agricultural products are the best, but can prove to be cost prohibitive, and may not be available in every store. Wherever and whenever it is possible, just peal the fruits and vegetables before using them. Another important step should be taken and practiced and that is to avoid consumption of processed foods, drugs, and cosmetics. All toxic chemicals, heavy metals, chlorine smelling water, processed foods, fat from the animal products, and the Trans fatty acids are very dangerous for all of us, especially for the stroke and heart patients.

LOSS OF WEIGHT, dieting, lack of activity, medication, and depression, etc. cause dryness of skin, wrinkles, loss of energy and strength, reduced and battered self image, etc. There is no single pill which will cure all these health handicaps instantly. One needs to consume the right foods, think clean and positively, and work at getting rid of such depressing health condition. This opens up the subject of combining foods to maximize the intake of right nutrients while not eating too much. There are so many combinations of foods that are available throughout the world. Older cultures had devised economical yet nutritious food combinations over times, which served the needs of body involved in a laborious, hard, and economically poor life style.

WRINKLES in the skin appear as we age, and especially if we suffer from stroke or heart attack and get on a special diet. Collagen is found in Brewer's yeast, peanuts, dried peas, nuts, sunflower and sesame seeds, wheat germ, olives avocados, and some other plant foods. Once these plant foods are combined with fruits and vegetable containing vitamin C, the benefic affect and the absorption of Collagen is enhanced tremendously. This combination of foods can improve cardio vascular function, cerebral circulation, protect against cellular degeneration of neurons in the brain, and in general optimal functioning of the brain. Collagen in combination with vitamin C is healthful for the skin which is the largest organ of the body. With this combination tightness of skin will be experienced, and the roughness of the skin will increasingly diminish over a period of time. Combine COLLAGEN containing foods with Vitamin C containing foods which are citrus fruits, strawberries, tomatoes, broccoli, Brussels sprouts, cabbage, green peppers, potatoes, sweet potatoes, kale, collards, mustard greens, etc. Practice various combinations of foods according to your taste, availability, and circumstances.

BRAIN AGING happens when it loses or depletes cell reserves. After the stroke or heart attack, it is quite common to have cell depletion in the brain. The population of dead cells increase, and when it is combined with the biological process which breaks down cells, tissues and molecules through oxidation, free radicals are created in the brain. Dead cells, tissues, and molecules are waste substances resulting from molecular degeneration, and need to be moved out of the brain for its healthy function. Vitamin E containing wheat germ mixed with fruits and vegetables, nuts, whole grains, yogurt, in varied combinations can help flush the waste out of the brain. Brain cells need nourishment on daily basis, and this feeding is crucial for the brain to function adequately, and to avoid senility prematurely. About 100,000 brain cells die each day. To slow down the death rate, as well as to maintain production of new cells each day require protein feeding to the brain. As long as it is possible, we should see that the cells in our body keep on replicating and forming new ones each day. When the cells stop replicating, or the replicating process slows down, we notice aging symptoms all over our body, including the slow down of the brain function. Depressing? I remember looking at my body with wrinkles on every joint and neck, arms, knees, stomach, and other places. No matter, what I tried but they would not go away. Yes, after 8 years, most wrinkles went away while I have been growing older. Avoid first or second stroke or heart attack with healthy food combinations of your own choice.

HORMONES

Hormones play a key role in replication and production of cells in our body. Hormones build walls and the inner components of cells. All glands secrete moisture which is mostly protein suitable for the body cells to ingest. This moisture is called hormones which are fed to billions of cells and tissues in our body. This process of hormone feeding to body cells and tissues creates and promotes replication and regeneration of cells, which is absolutely necessary to offset the cell decay and aging process, at least to some extent. There are several glands which require regular supply of protein for adequate health and functioning. Hence, protein in our diet becomes essential for the adequate supply of hormones in our body, which in fact promotes the youthfulness in our physical and mental self. Glands and hormones are mostly protein. All glands in our body work in harmony in relation to each other. If one gland is functioning inadequately, then all other glands become sluggish and less than adequate in function. Therefore, harmony among glands is essential. This essential harmony among glands can easily be accomplished by moderate, regular and sustainable physical activity which employs all body functions like household work, gardening, farming, playing a sport, aerobics, etc. There are many glands in our body, but the most prominent ones are:

THYROID GLAND, located at the base of the throat in front of the wind pipe, uses protein from our daily diet and, in return, produces Thyroxin, an important hormone. Thyroxin regulates the consumption of food in our body, usage of oxygen, rate at which our bodies process the food and the metabolism in general. It provides protein nourishment to body cells and tissues, and moistens the skin to give it a younger appearance. It is a kind of rejuvenating hormone. Lack or insufficient quantities of Thyroxin, can cause a condition called hypothyroid which could make our brains to slow down, make us look older prematurely, adversely affect the digestive system, tiredness and other related symptoms may appear. To feed your brain and put some gusto in the body, it is recommended that protein be taken in combination with vegetables containing iodine. There are some ocean fish that are high in protein and iodine, but that could be expensive as well as may contain other undesirable substances due to chemical and toxic pollution in the environment. Again, this combination will stimulate the brain, and may help prevent strokes.

PITUITARY GLAND, at the base of the brain, also called the master gland, uses protein to produce about 9 hormones to stimulate hypothalamus. One of the hormones produced in this chain process is ACTH which is known to create a defense mechanism against arthritis. ACTH is also known to stimulate the adrenal gland to produce various hormones like hydrocortisone which is a natural arthritis defense. Hormones produced by pituitary gland control, to a great extent, the muscles, skeleton, tendons, etc. Combination of plant protein and animal protein is an adequate way to feed the pituitary gland which produces at least nine hormones which help the patient to strengthen the tendons, muscles, body in general.

ADRENAL GLANDS, located next to the kidneys, produce hormone known as adrenalin. Adrenalin provides a kind of instant alert the nerves and muscles in the body. It helps build up and sharpen the reflexes. It is the hormone which alerts the body instantly. It improves vision, hearing, nerves, heart, muscles, removal of toxins, stress, etc. A combination of protein foods mixed with vitamin C containing foods is recommended to feed the adrenal glands.

PANCREAS, located behind the lower section of the stomach, like sweetbread in animals, produces hormone known as Insulin. Insulin helps the blood to convert sugar as it is needed by the body. Insulin production must be adequate and consistent, so that the exact amount of sugar is provided to the body. Consuming too much fat and sugar, and not enough protein, leads to weakness of pancreas which then fails to produce adequate insulin to regulate the blood sugar. When sugar does not get burned and regulated, diabetes sets in, thereby resulting in excessive thirst, unhealed wounds, obesity, cardio vascular disease, etc. Besides, reducing fat and sugars in the diet, adequate nourishment needs to be provided to pancreas to continuously produce insulin. A combination of protein from animal and plant source and carbohydrates from vegetables is recommended.

The **SEX GLANDS**, female sex glands are ovaries located in the lower region of women, which makes it possible to reproduce and give birth. Male sex gland is prostate glad which is located just below the bladder. Female sex glands produce two hormones: estrogen and progesterone which provide women the fertility and the pretty and delicate looks. A combination of animal protein, plant protein, and vegetables is recommended for adequate supply of estrogen and progesterone.
In males, prostate gland produces hormone known as testosterone which produces vigor, vitality, and fertility. Lack of this hormone in the male body may cause enlargement of prostate gland, sterility, etc. which, in turn, affect the brain adversely and cause depression. A combination of raw vegetable and fruits with fat free animal protein is recommended.

PARATHYROID GLANDS, total 4 in number, located around the thyroid gland just in front of the wind pipe. Parathyroid glands produce hormone known as parathormone which helps to regulate the use of phosphorus and calcium in the body. Lack of sufficient parathormone in the body may cause nervous instability, uncontrollable rage and anger, sudden outbursts, and other emotional irregularities. A combination of foods containing protein, calcium, and phosphorous is recommended.

THYMUS GLAND, located just below thyroid gland at the base of neck, produces a number of hormones which stimulate the metabolism of minerals, calcium, and phosphorous. Thymus hormones feed the brain with protein, and protect it from senility. Thymus hormones manufacture white blood corpuscles which become a natural guard against infections.

These hormones also build and repair red blood cells which aid in the healing process. Most definitely, they improve mental alertness which a stroke patient needs. A combination of grains, wheat germ, and fruits is recommended for a healthy thymus.

The best advice that I had received, many years ago, was to eat less amount of protein each day. In order to do that I had to learn to recognize the sources of protein in my food, and then I started to reduce the quantities of protein, especially the dense ones which are found in animal products. I started to eat a moderate amount of fish per weak, moderate amount of tofu more often, beans and lentils, regularly. Further, I reduced the portions of my daily intake of food. I felt better.

ALCOHOL

Do you know that a moderate amount of ALCOHOL, preferably in the form of red wine, is good for the body? Researchers around the world along with Dr. Michael Mogadam believe that any kind of alcohol is good for the body as long as the consumption is around 2 drinks per day. Alcohol reduces the risk of stroke and heart attacks, it reduces blood clotting. Some alcoholic drinks contain antioxidants like catechin and quercetin which help reduce the oxidation of LDL and HDL cholesterols in the body. One to two glasses of red wine helped me relax and digest my meals more easily. It increases the levels of good cholesterol (HDL) in the body, if taken in moderation. However, excessive use of alcohol can be bad for stomach lining, liver, and could inhibit omega-3 fatty acids absorption. For most purposes, red and white wines are both beneficial to stroke and heart patients, however, red grapes with which the red wine is made of contains a unique antioxidant known as resveratrol. Resveratrol is the most affective antioxidant to reduce oxidation of LDL cholesterol.

TEA

There is one drink that has gained acceptability from almost all nutritionists, and that is TEA. Every now and then nutritionists rediscover the good foods and drinks that have been adopted for thousands of years by Chinese and Indians. Tea, green or black, is good for you, because it contains several antioxidants. It has been advised that the best way to benefit from drinking tea is without sugar or milk mixed in it. However, there are benefits to be received even if you decide to mix in sugar and milk in your tea. There are two antioxidants in tea that are very special in reducing the risk of stroke and heart attack. These antioxidants are: Quercetin, and Catechin. Also, tea is very good for the bladder, because it flushing out the viruses and bacteria from the bladder.

CHOCOLATE

There is another great source of antioxidants and that is chocolate / cocoa. Chocolate is rich in antioxidants, vitamins A & B, iron, calcium, potassium, phosphorus, copper, Chocolate contains Phenythelamine which is a great stimulant for the brain. Phenythelamine is the ingredient in chocolate that provides the sense of pleasure to the brain. People of France have wine and chocolate as essentials for daily food intake, and probably that could be an important reason for them to live the longest in the world. Besides its pleasure giving attributes, it reduces the oxidation of LDL cholesterol, however, if it is consumed in excess may prove to be less beneficial but rather harmful.

PHYTOCHEMICALS

There are some chemicals in various foods, which provide color, aroma and unique fragrance to them. These chemicals are known as PHYTOCHEMICALS, and they are biologically active. Phytochemicals do not have any nutritional value, but they do provide resistance against disease to plants. These chemicals are fat free and do not contain any calories, and the medical community does not consider them to be 'essentials'. How-ever, there are some members of the medical community who do think that Phytochemicals could save our lives. Dr. Laurie Deutsch Mozian believes that Phytochemicals can help prevent and treat a variety of dis-eases like Cardio Vascular Disease, cancer, menopause, PMS, osteoporosis, prostate problems, and many more. Then there are other parts of plants which are labeled as PHYTONUTRIENTS which are biologically active, and are 'essentials' for sustaining life

FREE RADICALS are singular molecules, who roam around to pair up with other molecules. Quite often, these free radicals attack the cells to pair up with their molecules, and this act can result in disease of some kind. Phytochemicals that act like antioxidants save the cells from such attacks by rushing to the site of attack and offering themselves to get paired up. This is a kind of sacrifice to save the cells. A large number of antioxidants in the body will prevent free radicals to attack body cells suc-cessfully. However, if antioxidants are in insufficient numbers, free radicals would be able to attack the cells successfully, resulting in decaying of cells and premature aging. There are hundreds, possibly thousands, of phy-tochemicals known to science, and they serve the body in number of ways. Some of them are: Carotenids (family of over 450 phytochemicals), is found in leafy vegetables, red and orange fruits. Isoflavones are found mostly in beans and tofu. Isoprenoids are mostly found in citrus fruits, carrots, cherries, and whole grains. Monoterpenes are found in citrus fruits, cherries, caraway, dill, and spearmint. Phytosterols are found mostly in peanuts, seeds, and some other nuts. Protease Inhibitors are found in chick peas, kidney beans, Brussels sprout, broccoli, spinach, corn, seeds, whole grains, potatoes, etc. All vegetables, fruits, nuts, seeds, and herbs contain some type of phytochemical/s, which brings us to the fact estab-lished thousands of years ago that in order to stay healthy and prevent dis-ease, one must eat vegetables and fruits of all colors and range, accompanied by all kinds of beans, seeds, nuts, and herbs.

This takes us to another phase of diet to prevent Stroke and cardio vascular disease. We have briefly covered the fats, cholesterol, AA/EPA ratio, vitamins, phytochemicals, etc. It will be very difficult for any one to cover all the good and healing nutrition and avoid all the bad things in one's daily meals. Clinically proven packaged health food intake will not prove to be practical, nor feasible. There are so many nutritional values we want and the sources are numerous, yet we should be able to enjoy the food we eat. Before we can enjoy the food, we have to like it. Each of us have individual taste, metabolism, family history, life style, work habits, physical activity range, financial and social scenario, environment, stress levels, etc. Therefore, we will end up doing the best we can under the given circumstances. If we can do as best as we can, then we are on the right track. Once we familiarize ourselves as to what is good for us, then we will end up making choices which can turn in to habits a little later. The reinforcement of good things in our food choices will definitely make a great difference. In between, we are bound to stray once in a while, and that is alright.

NON VEGETARIANS should develop, if they already have not, a taste and liking for foods which are prepared in combination of several vegetables, beans, grains, fruits, and herbs. There are almost limitless options to suit individual taste buds. You should be able to make your own recipe according to your own taste, availability of types of foods, and budget. Visit various eating places, and start looking at different preparations in the light of healthy diet. You will come up with several recipes that you would like to try at home. Learn to enjoy preparing your own favorite meals, no matter how simple they might be. It will be a source of concentration, occupation, creativity, continuous improvisation, skill, and joy. This can turn out to be a great hobby which will feed your body for many decades to come.

Just for hints, try combining lean or non fat protein foods with vegetables, nuts, and fruits, in small portions in a single meal. If it is not possible for one reason or another then try to achieve this balance by extending it to the whole day. Try to taste as many vegetables, fruits, nuts, seeds, beans, etc. as you possible can, of course in very small quantities. Prevent cardio vascular disease by incorporating phytochemicals in your daily diet. It is impossible to eat all the good things that nature provides us to consume to stay healthy, however, we can key phytochemical rich foods in our daily diets. Foods rich in monounsaturated fatty acids, soluble fiber which are found in oats and beans; allicin which is found in garlic; folic acid, vitamin B6 and vitamin B3 found in certain fish, bananas, baked potatoes, soy beans, oranges, sunflower seeds, and flax seeds; pectin which is found in apples, lentils, spinach, broccoli, brewer's yeast, broccoli, oranges; flavonoids as found in purple grape juice; capsicum as found in red peppers; eritadenine as found in shiitake mushrooms; antioxidants as found in green and processed tea; There are many other phytochemicals that provide our body the protective support. Everything that grows in this world has some benefit for out body.

GROOM YOURSELF and dress well every day. You are living your life, and you want to look best every day of the week. Create a routine and live with it. This will provide you with the control you need to prevent stroke or heart attack occurrence in the future. Once a week give your hair a super treatment with mayonnaise by covering your head with it and then letting it stay there for 20 to 30 minutes, before you shampoo. Similarly, give your face a face lift by applying a mixer of an egg, cucumber with peel, and heavy cream. Mix them well in a machine and then put the mixture in the refrigerator for some time to evaporate. Leave this paste on your face and around upper neck area for half an hour. You will see wrinkled and dried out skin will begin to clear out in a few weeks time. You may want to try some other method of enhancing your hair health and facial health with which you are more familiar or the ones that are more convenient for you.

Learn the **HEALTH HISTORY OF YOUR FAMILY** which should encompass all the females and males in your father's family, and similarly all the males and females in your mother's family. This will provide you with the genetic pattern of health events that may affect you. Eventually, genetic pattern of health will determine the health events in your life, no matter how careful you can be with your diet and life style. You can delay such health events in your life, but cannot get out of it, until current biological research scientists find out a way to successfully manipulate the individual genes in our body. Now the key element of learning the family health history is recognition of symptoms of such health events. First hand knowledge of your own health will provide you the capabilities to recognize earliest symptoms of the family diseases. This is one of the reasons I stress that in every health event, we must take control of our health and manage it from the beginning to the end. You must know each developing stages of even a common cold. Once you become completely familiar with all the stages and symptoms, it will become quite easy to avoid getting a cold altogether. While the word common cold is in the picture, it is important to know that having more than three colds per year is a serious matter for the stroke and heart attack patient. Do whatever you can to avoid colds, and definitely influenza. If possible and if it is the recommendation of your doctor then do take the flue shots each year. If the specific symptoms of family disease are recognized, there exists a high probability that you will be able to avert it completely, or at least postpone it. Genes are programmed to produce certain milligrams of cholesterols naturally for the adequate and healthy function of the body. However, if the family history indicates that after the age of 50 years, most family members suffered cardio vascular disease due to high cholesterols, whether self induced by eating excessive amounts of fatty foods, etc., or not, the probability of your body to show similar pattern of high blood cholesterol will be high once you cross the age of 50 years. But you can change this pattern through self awareness, recognition of early symptoms, regular check ups, discipline, and the management of your well being by yourself.

DANGERS TO AVOID

Although, we all need to be careful of RADIATION, however, for a patient it becomes much more important to avoid lengthy exposure to it. Ultra-violet rays have big wave length, and regularly sustained exposure to it can damage the DNA in the skin cells, and can cause cataracts in the eyes. So just be careful whether you are a patient or not; it can happen to any one. But why should a stroke or heart patient bear another burden when there are enough to deal with on hourly basis each day. High tension cable towers, microwave towers, power generators, electrical transformers, nuclear power plants, etc. do produce various kinds of radiation at different wave lengths, and living or working in the vicinity may not be healthy for a stroke or heart patient. There is another kind of **RADIATION** which has short wave length. This radiation is highly dangerous. It is the same radiation which emanates from a nuclear explosion and operating x-ray machines. This radiation of short wave length can knock electrons from DNA, and make them ionized which can give room to a host of other health problems for the stroke patient to face in near future. Higher doses of this radiation of short wave length can damage the immune system. It includes all kinds of x-rays. Avoid unnecessary and excessive exposure to x-rays, as much as you can manage to help. Avoid its accumulative effects. For now, we do not have to discuss the effects of this kind of radiation that emanates from the nuclear explosion. Plenty of fruits and vegetables in the daily diet may block the chemical reaction that leads to the injury to DNA, but there is no guarantee. However, do make an effort to avoid heating pads, electric blankets, electric clocks, computer screens, and damaged microwave ovens, Microwave foods only in ceramics or glass utensils. Never use plastic containers in the microwave ovens, because use of plastic can introduce foreign molecules in the food. Do not live near the Microwave Transmitter, or in the path of Military Communication site. Regarding on going research and emerging developments do consult your doctor and seek advice.

To get better and to remain healthy, patients should avoid **DEHYDRATION** which can be especially dangerous for older stroke and heart patients. When we are young, our bodies contain about 90% of water, and this water content of our bodies keep falling in percentage as we grow older. Among elderly persons water content falls to 60%, or even lower. Water acts as an insulator. When it is cold outside, water content in our body acts like an insulator, thereby minimizing the heat loss and maintaining the suitable temperature of body. On the other hand when it is hot outside, water keeps us relatively cool by maintaining the suitable temperature of body. Dehydration can cause kidney problems like: infections, stones, etc. To combat these kidney problems, patients have to take medication which, in turn, puts extra burden of kidneys, because the medication will end up passing through the kidneys. Also, lack of water makes the blood much thicker than normal. Kidneys are subjected to enormous pressure to pass thick blood which has to pass through the kidneys to get rid of body waste. Urine should be pale yellow, and if it is darker, then personal physician must be consulted. In order to avoid all these unpleasant experiences and uncertain outcomes, stroke and heart patients are recommended to drink a lot of water which can keep their system flushed on daily basis.

It is quite common for the stroke and heart patients to experience IRREGULARITY in bowel movement. Lack of ability to move freely, general weakness of the limbs, trauma, confusion, and incapacity to carry out most tasks compels the patient to be confined and sedentary. Such a condition makes it obvious for the patient to develop constipation, and suffer the related consequences which could prove to be disastrous. The most common response for most people, stroke patients and non stroke patients, is to take some laxative to deal with **CONSTIPATION**. Stroke and heart attack patients should avoid taking laxatives. Laxatives may prove to be comforting in the sense of emptying the stomach, but at the same time, laxatives empty the body of minerals. All minerals are precious to our body. Calcium is the most important mineral in our body. Without calcium, and with the depletion of calcium, stroke and heart patients, as well as others, will experience a well known condition known as osteoporosis. Lack of calcium compels the body to take calcium from our bones for the daily function of the body, which makes our bones less dense. This results in bone loss, shrinkage of body structure, bone loss in the jaw and roots of teeth, loss of teeth, bones get broken easily, etc. Do not hesitate to discuss these matters with your physician.

Therefore avoid commercial laxatives whenever it is possible. Instead, consume bran, natural fiber containing beans, vegetables, and fruits, which are natural laxatives and do not empty the body of precious minerals, especially calcium. It is a well known fact that without vitamin D, calcium does not get absorbed in the body. Therefore, taking vitamin D on a daily bases, is crucial for the stroke and heart patients to be able to absorb calcium. It is also known that our skin produces vitamin D when exposed to the ultraviolet light in the sunshine. Younger skin can perform this production of vitamin D quite efficiently, but unfortunately the older skin fails to produce similar results. Kidney and Gall Bladder diseases are also the cause of vitamin D deficiency. Daily exposure to the sunshine is highly recommended. For those who are unable to expose themselves to sunshine on daily basis, vitamin D supplements are recommended. If you are taking fiber in a capsule form, then make sure that you consume a lot of water with it, because fiber alone would not move the bowels. Fiber's action is dependent upon water which must be consumed at least 12 glasses a day. Prunes and figs are also recommended for daily consumption for relief from CONSTIPATION.

Besides all the remedies, there is a stomach exercise which may be beneficial for the stroke or heart patient in more than one way. This exercise is similar to the exercise recommended for incontinence, which is to squeeze the pelvic muscle and release it after a few seconds, which will help develop the pelvic muscle and the control over it. To avoid CONSTIPATION and the food getting lodged in the intestinal track, just try to squeeze the stomach so that you can see small cavity is formed on each side of the stomach. Bulk of stomach will gather in the middle forming a ridge like shape. Squeezing, holding for a few seconds in that position, and then releasing it would build and strengthen certain stomach muscles which may aid proper bowel movement. If you can perform this exercise then probably you are not over weight, and are in good shape.

Stroke and heart patients with swollen legs, painful stiffness in knees and ankles may incorporate vitamin C containing foods. Such foods will prove to be very beneficial. Alternatively, vitamin C supplements should be taken on regular basis. Some patients experience dryness of the mouth caused by lack of saliva in the mouth. Stroke and heart patients do want to minimize their health problems and most definitely do not wish to add on more problems. Saliva has anti-bacterial effect that not only protects the inside of the mouth from various infections, but also protects the teeth. Lack of saliva can be resulted due to many reasons, but the prominent one is the drugs that patients are subjected to take. Anti-depressants, anti-hypertension, tranquilizers, etc. happen to be the most common cause of dryness of the mouth. Consultation with the personal physician to reduce the intake of drugs should be considered.

Stroke and heart attack patients and the non patients who suddenly experience total **BLINDNESS** or blindness in a part of vision field should take notice of the fact that a blood clot may be blocking the flow of blood to the eye/s or to its nerve connection. This is a warning of an impending stroke. Visual loss varies from a small blind spot to total blindness which may last a few minutes to several minutes. Cholesterol deposit (atherosclerosis) can limit or block the supply of blood to the retina artery, which can cause blindness for few minutes or longer. If the clot dissolves or breaks up and the blood supply resumes, then the vision returns. If the blindness prolongs then a physician must be consulted immediately. However, in the meantime you can help yourself by gently massaging the upper eyelid of closed eye, with on and off gentle pressure with a soft towel. This gentle massage for a minute or two may disperse the blood clot and bring back your vision. Other exercises that I practiced were eye ball movements from one corner to another, up and down, and side ways, on a regular basis. At one time, I could not see the print in the newspapers and magazines. I had to bring the printed material very close to my eyes in a bright light to be able to read it. I needed eye glasses for sure. But, I could not visualize myself wearing glasses every day, and be dependent on them. I was vein as well. After regular exercises, now I am able to read the printed material, and I do not use eye glasses. In fact, most of the time my vision is better now than it was a few years before experiencing strokes.

Be aware of **SALT** consumption. Salt is known as Sodium Chloride and its value is mentioned on each food label that is pasted on the processed foods. Its chemical symbol is "Na" which is abbreviation of Latin word "natrium". Monosodium Glutamate, baking soda, baking powder, soft drinks, club soda, beer, deserts, puddings, anti-acids, some breakfast cereals, various processed foods, cheeses, and some non-prescription drugs, etc. contain high levels of salt. Intake of high levels of salt from young age onward is harmful, and can cause permanent high blood pressure later in life. Many of us could develop hypertension and cardio vascular disease by continually taking high levels of salt in our foods.

Most of the harmful salt intake is from the consumption of commercially prepared foods which are generally loaded with above normal levels of salt. Just like anything else, each individual responds to salt intake differently. Genes regulate the specific response to salt in the body. Too much salt can cause hypertension, excessive urination, etc. Hypertension can lead to stroke or heart attack, while excessive urination can lead to depletion of calcium from the body. Depletion of calcium from the body results in osteoporosis. On the other hand, if salt intake is significantly reduced, it can cause adverse effects to some people. Decreased quantity of salt intake may lead to higher blood triglycerides, lower HDL, and stiffness of arteries. Also lack of iodine in the salt may cause thyroid problems. So, there is balance of salt intake for every individual to maintain good health.

Some researchers believe that stroke and heart patients should be careful in using **ANTIHISTAMINE** and decongestants which are generally prescribed as cold remedies. Antihistamine dries up the nasal secretion, and decongestant shrinks blood vessels in the lining of nose. It may be useful relief for an average person; however, it is dangerous for a stroke or heart patient and also for the individuals who are suffering from hypertension / high blood pressure. Shrinking of blood vessels in the nasal lining may also result in shrinking of blood vessels elsewhere in the body. Stroke, heart patients, and hypertensive persons are already prone to contracting of blood vessels significantly, and if combined with the use of decongestants, blood pressure may climb to an unsafe level. This drug induced high blood pressure can cause strokes from bleeding in the brain, and heart attacks. Patients and non patients with high blood pressure should seek the advice of their physician in respect to using antihistamines and decongestants.

Since high **BLOOD PRESSURE** or hypertension play an important part in predicting, monitoring, and curing cardio vascular disease, accuracy of blood pressure reading becomes essential. Many, who have been diagnosed with high blood pressure, may instead have false hypertension. Subjects with the condition of hardening of arteries may clock a higher blood pressure. Also, if the blood pressure measuring instrument is too hard on the arm then the outcome could also be a higher blood pressure reading. This higher blood pressure reading is, in fact, related to diastolic pressure (lower reading). The systolic (upper reading) pressure is not affected by the hardness of the measuring instrument on the arm. Diastolic pressure (lower) is the important one for anti-hypertension treatment. If the blood pressure readings are taken with a smaller cuff which is too small for the arm then the readings are going to be elevated. A small cuff on a large arm can produce results which will show high blood pressure, when the person could just be having normal blood pressure. This unintended error may result in normal person taking high blood pressure medication unnecessarily. On a few occasions I and some friends took the blood pressure readings on various machines and almost each reading was a bit different than the one just taken a few minutes before. Some good doctors take at least two readings of blood pressure on the patient's arrival to determine an accurate level. Also, who calibrates the blood pressure taking instruments? Could it be possible that the measuring device gets damaged after some usage, or there is a percentage of defective products to start with? Yet there is another circumstance when the blood pressure readings could prove to be erroneous and, that is, when person is nervous while in doctor's office and under going blood pressure test. I have always been nervous during my visits to the doctor's office, and quite many people are. All these scenarios suggest that a lot of people could be taking high blood pressure medicine when, in fact, they do not require.

So, **ACCURATE READING** of blood pressure is quite important especially for the stroke and heart patients who may consider attending to a few factors before and during such readings. Blood pressure readings will rise if coffee or tobacco were consumed just before the test. Therefore, do not consume coffee or tobacco, etc. for at least two hours before the blood test. Blood pressure should be taken from both arms, primarily because there may be an abnormal artery in one arm which can produce false blood pressure reading. The arm should be in a resting position on the table during blood pressure testing. If the arm is hanging lose, without any support or rest, the test may show high blood pressure when, in fact, it is not the case. Patients, who are under treatment for high blood pressure, should stand during the blood pressure testing. You will find a drop in blood pressure reading when it is taken while you are standing, and this may relieve you of the burden of having to take medication when you do not need to. The correct blood pressure reading also depends upon your activity level just before the test. If you have been walking or exercising before, just rest 20 to 30 minutes before the test for its accuracy which is essentially beneficial for you. High blood pressure causes strokes and heart attacks, therefore, it must be controlled. Avoiding consumption of salt, optimizing consumption of calcium, regular intake of potassium, meditation, walking, socializing, mind and life style balance, and visiting your doctor, etc. will help you to bring down the blood pressure.

ACCURACY IN BLOOD TESTS

Blood tests play a very important role in doctor's decision making at each step from prior to diagnoses, to prognosis and recovery. Blood test is a must for the stroke and heart patients, and not too many really understand the print out of such tests. We must acquaint ourselves about the 'kind' of blood test the doctor ordered, as there are many kinds, and what was the outcome of it. If we understand those results, then we can take voluntary steps to rectify the problem in conjunction with doctor's advice and medication. Patients will be surprised how fast they recover by self participation in the healing process. Also, this active self participation will ensure that the tests were conducted on your blood, and the tests do not belong to someone else. Of course, there are several variables of time, day, state of mind for the past few days, digestion, etc but they are not too significant in determining the accuracy of blood tests. The accuracy of blood tests are crucial, because inaccuracy will take the patient to a treatment which is not required for the patient's health condition.

Our **PERSONALITY** plays a significant role in the management of stroke and heart disease, and also avoidance of such occurrences in the future. This personality trait is not universal, but is present in some people. People with an innate urge to challenge other people, compete and want to be the first, aggressive in sports and in discussions, want to have the last word, want to win only, hate to lose, generally aggressive and hostile are more prone to having strokes and heart attacks. I know this personality well, because I possess it. Everyone in my parents' side of the family had it and all suffered from cardio vascular disease. Such aggressive and somewhat hostile people have been classified as "type 'A' personality". Some researchers believe that such type A personality people have hormonal abnormalities which, in turn, raise cholesterol in their blood. Again, increased cholesterol in the blood induces more blood clotting which progresses to blood vessels resulting in stroke or heart attack much earlier in life.

To counter this kind of behavior, we must develop a personality which accepts that we are not going to be the winners in every game we play, every discussion we get involved in, and everyone else happens to be a competitor. We should learn to accept losing in a healthy way. A happy and congenial loser is the term most commonly used in sports arena. Some quiet thinking will help us to recognize that all winnings come to an end one time or another. There is always going to be a better sports person, or a stronger person around the corner.

Losing should not be viewed as the end of the world. Better circumstances will always present themselves from time to time. Every human being is a winner in some ways which makes him or her happy and satisfied to a certain degree. Everyone in this world is an achiever one way or another. It seems that contentment in life is equally distributed among all living creatures, that is, if we incorporate all the elements of life that constitute contentment. A stable and accommodating state of mind will lead all of us to accept others as winners when we lose. It is a great state of mind, because it raises the self esteem in us. Having self esteem gives us self confidence, self control, and acceptability. Self esteem in conjunction with respect for others and acceptance of inevitability of outcomes from events in lifetime will take a patient a long way to early recovery from the effects of stroke or heart attack. To some extent giving up a lot of receivables and some valuables, and the acceptance of it helped me get better, relearn most essentials to run daily life, and to move on.

There are other personality traits and social conditions that are important for the patients and non patients to note, and they are: INSOMNIA, tired on awakening, delving on work related or inter personal issues before going to bed and trying to come up with self serving solutions, getting angry under stress and also getting angry when things don't happen the intended way, etc. Light exercise, amusing activities, humor, and letting the chips fall where they may could help to counter these conditions. It has also been known that males and females who find difficulties in getting along with other people, who are single, and who have family troubles are at a greater risk of having a stroke and heart attack, or recurring one if they have already had one. Interaction with a variety of people of all ages could resolve this condition. Again, stroke persons should be in normal social environment where all kinds of people of all ages exist. Patients should minimize their presence in the community where several patients with various disabilities are gathered. Such an atmosphere may be good for camaraderie, exchange of sympathies and prescription news, ventilation of aggravations relative to medical help, etc., but it could also become a comfort zone and routine which may delay the timely recuperation. The patient may not want to leave such an environment and may receive an equally acceptable response from the medical help people. After all, provision of healthcare is a business for profit. Relearning everything is the main objective of the stroke patient, and it should be kept in mind all the time so that appropriate actions could be taken.

After the first stroke and the subsequent strokes which took place after a few months, one after another, I became remarkably aware of the fact that my upper and lower LIPS were not in complete alignment. Either my lower jaw had shifted to one side or the upper jaw. My hearing was not the best. I had difficulty to speak, and difficulties to move my tongue freely. To chew food and to swallow it felt quite strange and difficult. Vision was greatly reduced, and with difficulty whatever I saw did not make any sense to me. In short I could not see the printed matter unless I brought it just a few inches from my eyes, and whatever I saw I failed to recognize. I could not recognize the English LANGUAGE, but I could somewhat understand the spoken word. All these faculties are very close to the brain which controls them in every way. They were damaged. This accumulative damage was the result of at least 3 strokes, possibly in different parts of the brain, inside a year. Circumstances and possibly my personality compelled me to correct my weaknesses, resulted from stroke/s, because I wanted to survive, get on my feet, and resume my life again. There was a substantial amount of ignorance and arrogance on my part. Ignorance, because I did not know the symptoms of stroke, and all the rules of healthcare system, and the process I should have followed. Arrogance, because I wanted to beat all the odds in getting better on my own, and show the world that I could do it myself without the healthcare system. Both elements were negative.

To be able to understand English, I started to keep the TV on and listened to whatever was on at any given time. Even though I found it difficult to look at the TV for more than a few minutes at a time, I kept it on, nevertheless. It was an exercise in comprehension which did expand with more listening and watching. For a long time, perhaps a few years, it was difficult to retain anything watched on TV for more than a minute or two. I learned to apply different methods for me to retain TV messages, and gradually I could remember messages and scenes for a much longer time. Initially, I watched the shows I was interested in, which motivated me and kept me focused. I watched old movies which I used to see when I was young, and there were more than a few on the TV. This was a great help. I started to remember the names of the stars, movies, and remembered scenes. This not only improved my English, memory, comprehension, hearing, vocabulary, but also diverted my attention from the painful issues of life which were the reasons of tension, let downs, aggravated, high blood pressure, anger which led to strokes. At that time, I thought I was speaking correctly, even though I found it difficult to speak and find the right words to complete a sentence, but somehow others were either walking away from me, or hanging up the phone on me. These were the same people who were my friends, business partners, neighbors, and acquaintances. How could anyone learn to speak correctly again without having someone to participate with? I started to sing whenever I could in my apartment. I used to feel aggravated when someone did not understand me. But somehow I got there where I could make a general conversation for a few minutes. You can do the same if you are not doing it currently, because it will empower you to manage your recuperation. If you are able to converse then you will be able to participate in life and be able to deal with the medical community quite effectively.

I remember attending a meeting with the Maryland State officials to obtain a certification, and this was after a couple of years from the series of stroke experience. The meeting took place in a board room with a number of other officials. The director asked me a couple of questions which I could not understand at all, and finally he asked me if I had any questions. My response was "what about". He asked me again if I wanted to ask him anything about the certification in question, and my response was "what questions"? "What do you want me to ask"? And possibly some other stupid remarks were made by me. I was not hearing correctly, and I did not comprehend correctly, and therefore I was finding difficulties to respond correctly. Also, without being able to understand completely what others are saying, and at the same time inability to speak properly, and not being able to express, all lead to irritation and anger. Irritation and anger are a complete "no" for a stroke or a heart patient. Sometimes, it leads the patient to frustration because with the concerted efforts to speak and understand the stroke patient is not likely to learn all that was lost in a short period of time.

Again, balance in the relearning process, activity, and expectations will be required for healthy recovery. Recovery achievements should be consistent and in small steps at a time. Efforts and expectations for speedy recovery will most likely lead to irritability, anger, and a disgusted state of mind. Such outcomes and feelings should be avoided, because they bring the patient to a state of helplessness, failure, self pity, doom and gloom, etc. Stroke and heart patients need tranquility, some accomplishments each day, activity, encouragement, day light, acceptability, accommodation, sincere care and some affection.

I remember picking up a written document, and failed to recognize the English language. Not only the vision was impaired but complete recognition of the English language was denied by the damaged brain. That was scary. I forced myself everyday to view and try to read the written material as many times as I could manage each day. Thanks to the internet facility which helped me. I used to look at the written material at very close range for a very long time and failing to make any sense of it. Gradually, I succeeded in rekindling my memory and started to read the language, understand it, and speak it. A lot of errors were made on daily basis. Most crucial ones were the cultural ones. Human interaction is the key to surviving in this world, of business. This interaction requires a set of rules governed by culture, local or universal. I experienced making grave errors in just about every aspect of my life on daily basis. I experienced humiliation due to my errors, but today I am better off than before. All of these unpleasant experiences used to make me feel ashamed later, and I used to curse myself for being a part of it. After so many years, I still make some errors, feel humiliated, and curse myself later, but gradually on fewer occasions now. If you make errors and commit social blunders, just consider them to be a part of the equation and make every effort to live with this reality. The acceptance of this reality may provide you some humor in the interim, but it will help you heal faster. I recommend that patients should explore the use of internet, and most definitely look in to Web TV who offers internet service via TV.

REASONING and comparative analytical ability disappear after stroke occurrence. As I mentioned before, the grown up person is reduced to a child in many aspects. It takes very long to purchase anything for a variety of reasons but primarily due to lack of memory retention and processing its recently received information. Unless the retention of what was just received is prolonged a bit longer its processing becomes difficult if not impossible. Another kind of difficulty can confront when choice has to be made between two similar products. Being unable to make a decision, I used to either return home without it, or bought two similar products when I needed just one. Also, I was buying repeatedly the same things that I had already bought a few days before. Reasoning, comparative analysis, making choices and arriving at a decision, perceiving right and wrong, perceiving what is good for me and what is not, differentiating friend from a foe, timely recognition of stranger from a friend, cold weather from a hot one (for short period), and many other such mental responses can become challenging parts of your daily life. On several occasions while chopping vegetables, I stopped only after seeing blood on my fingers or hand. There were no pain signals. Therefore, the caregivers must make sure that the patient is completely free from such happenings. Ironically, if the patient delays in the participatory activities of life, the relearning process will be delayed much further. The best solution, in my opinion, is to let the patient do any and everything, which is extremely healthy and therapeutic for him or her, under a close supervision. Loved ones or caregivers should supervise stroke or heart attack patient as if he or she were their child who is going through the initial learning lessons of life.

READING and **WRITING** become equally difficult after the stroke. I went through the basics of reading and writing. Rest and gradual recuperation of lost memory helped me to read and write to a workable degree now. For reading, I had to develop focus, patience, energy, and interest which are not difficult. The difficult part is energy, vision, and the persistence. I learned reading and comprehension on the internet. It was easy to do so without any noise, questions, answers, etc. I learned reading on my own time at my own pace, and this improved my memory as well. Even to this day, I have the same routine in the morning each day. Stroke and heart patients lose energy to do most things, and to be able to relearn reading energy is required. Regular rest periods and positive outlook can help a lot. Writing becomes an entirely different challenge. Here, the stroke or heart attack patient needs the use of arm, hand, fingers, and finger tips, besides concentration. After the stroke, my finger tips, hand and the arm did not move in the way I had known before. I found them to be out of control. Finger tips were unable to hold the pen in the same position tightly enough to continue writing, and making the hand, wrist, and part of the arm travel in the direction of writing. It seemed that all the components of arm and the hand wanted to do their own thing, and there did not seem to be any proper coordination among them. Without a complete coordination of all the components involved writing skills cannot be regained. I overcame this disability by various light exercises involving finger tips, wrist, arm, and the shoulder, one at time, separately. I found a simple exercise rule: hold the pen tightly, write one word, then slightly move your wrist to the right and write the next word, and so on and so forth. This exercise helped me to start writing in legible manner, without pen streaking out in different directions, and also not being able to stay on a straight horizontal line. There is another aspect of writing difficulties is the element of missing words in a sentence. Even after about 10 years, I still forget to put "and", "to", "with", etc. while I am writing, and strangely I am never aware of it until much after when I read it again. During fatigued state, I make such omissions more often than otherwise. With a little practice on regular basis, one can relearn the writing skills, and progressively improve other areas of writing as the writing is practiced regularly.

For **SPEECH** improvement, I took speech therapy which helped me immensely. I was provided with the opportunity to listen to various words, in person, at a close range with correct phonetics. Correct hearing is essential to be able to speak correctly. For this, I was given a hearing test which revealed that I was unable to hear certain frequencies of sound waves. I was also advised that such a phenomenon was not uncommon among people above 60 years of age. Speech therapy did help me in recognizing the right phonetics, after practicing with the speech therapist, I learnt to pronounce the words correctly, or near correctly. One thing is definite in my thinking and, that is, never stop trying to speak, even if it feels difficult to do so. Also, never stop trying to speak even if other people are unable to comprehend and make any sense out of your words. Unless you speak and make errors, you are not going to relearn to speak. Children do it so easily because they do not feel shy, and the people around recognize and accept that they are children who are learning to speak. People around a stroke patient expect the patient to speak normally and behave appropriately because they know that you have learned speaking long before. People expect you to be able to speak properly, and when you do not they scoff at you and eventually abandon you. You feel sad and disheartened which takes you to the bin of depression. To overcome this, go to a coffee shop or shopping mall and listen to the people next to your table or bench while sipping your coffee. Exchange glances a few times, and sooner or later some conversation will take place. At this time, keep your conversation to the minimum. In response, say only those words that you can say properly and after that use smile and nod to fill the gaps. Other people may think that you have a tooth problem. So be it. Each day identify those words, sentences, and topics which can come out of your mouth without much difficulty. Try to rehearse these words and sentences. Hereafter, expand your domain by talking to people selectively. Very soon you will have set of words, sentences, and the topics of conversation which do not make you overly uncomfortable, and stay within the comfort zone. Expand this zone on a daily basis, and you will be surprised to see how many people start talking to you. Talking you need to do because without it you will not be able relearn it. If you create language or speech foul up, don't panic or feel humiliated. We, all do these things on regular basis even under completely normal and healthy conditions. Keep upgrading your level of conversation on a regular basis by adding new words and sentences with known topics. Go to the next step by socializing with those people who choose to talk to you. Buy them tea or coffee on a regular basis, or accept theirs. Moreover, in the relearning process you are receiving the skill at the price of humiliation. Make sure that you are not seeking pity by describing your health predicament to others. These others will abandon you or take advantage of you the moment they know you are stroke or heart patient and are in a difficult situation. Stay positive, confident, and determined to learn and you will succeed within a short period of time. You want to relearn to speak correctly, and there is no way any one should be able to stop you or discourage you from doing so, because you are managing your recovery, and are in control of this management. To relearn making conversation you will have to start speaking confidently, no matter how difficult it my be for others to comprehend.

Routine household tasks become a challenge, which have to be dealt with on hourly and daily basis, that is, if the stroke patient does not have any medical help, or a loved one to take care of. If you are by yourself and are faced to cope with the aftermath of a stroke occurrence, then follow the same method that I adopted, besides listening to your doctor's advice. Habitually, I used to complete all tasks in the house very expeditiously and then get involved in something else. After the stroke, I was unable to complete any task in one take, and even the attempt used to make me completely exhausted and useless thereafter. I adopted a method which worked. I used to brush my teeth and then take rest. After this when I was completely rested, I would shave at my own pace, and rest afterwards. In other words, I broke down most routines in to smaller bits, and accomplished each bit at my own time within my own energy levels. The only humorous part was the laundry. After the washing machine had stopped, I was supposed to put the clothes in to the dryer, but instead I used to look at the clothes and did not know the next step. Almost all the times, after transferring the washed clothes from the washer to the dryer, I kept on searching by running my hand for clothes that might have stuck to walls of the washer, repeatedly. Firstly, I could not receive and process the message which my eyes were witnessing, and secondly I could not retain the message that the task was completed. Looking back, it makes me laugh. I still end up doing the same thing, but very rarely.

I have started to believe that nature or the universe provides an aura of protection to all humans and other species. Unless we are determined to be suicidal and continually proceed in that direction, nature does protect us. Even after getting better and functional, I remember having just a few capsule of energy in my body, and once I spent those energy capsules I used to become somewhat lifeless and useless. I had marginal energy levels just to be able to finish a task or two, after which I needed rest. At such times, the judgment capabilities reach at a very low level. I remember on the way to home after visiting a business associate just for a few minutes when I felt tired, I had a feeling and a strange urge to drive through the empty space underneath the belly of flatbed tractor trailer. This experience in my mind was repeated on several occasions later under similar levels of tiredness and loss of energy. Judgment became so poor that part of the brain kept on considering to enter that empty space, Analyzing such mental experiences, I reached a definite conclusion that as a stroke patient with limited energy levels, I should minimize the number of tasks I perform within a given time frame. Also, since the mind keeps busy 24 hours a day, no matter what task is being performed, I should be at ease with myself and the world, and should not be carrying more than one or two thoughts in my mind during performing a particular task like driving.

Once, I was driving in a snow storm in the evening when ice had fallen and got impacted a few hours before. I was returning from a memorial of a dear friend who had recently died from drowning while scuba diving. I was carrying the thoughts of my young friend, concentrating on traffic, concentrating hard to stay within the groves created by traffic in the ice below the falling snow, and trying to see my path of driving in almost zero visibility, and at the same time I was nursing myself with the thoughts of being macho, brave, and accomplisher. Obviously, all this load of thoughts and concerns proved to be too much for my body and the freshly healed brain. At less than 45 MPH, my car made a 360 degree roundabout turn on the dark highway, and I thought I had it under control just for a moment only when the car skidded sideways in to the ditch below. Once again, nature was there to save my life but with a lesson. My car could not complete the upside turn because it was stopped by the dried branches of bushes and the trees; it was suspended on its side, and could not be seen or heard from the highway. Luckily, I came out of it alive and without any injuries, and came out on the highway to press 9 on my cell phone for the police, Surviving from this experience, I was reminded about the 100th time that just perform one task at time within the available scope of the energy capsule. I have been keeping this thought with me all the time and I immediately stop the activity or do not participate at all beyond the energy levels I have at a given time.

BITE ALIGNMENT of upper and lower teeth may be off in some stroke patients. When upper and lower jaws are not performing in a harmonious manner, then teeth tend to hit inner walls of the mouth. I experienced repeated bites at the same spot, and other times at different locations. These bites get infected which becomes a cause of constant pain, and certainly not good for the stroke patient. Stroke or heart patient does not need new problems. Slow munching and complete focus are the answers. Munching slowly is healthy, and helps digest food properly and timely. Also, eating slowly will strengthen jaw muscles and produce sufficient saliva to aid swallowing of food. Besides, well chewed food relieves the body of extra work, as well as enables it to extract nutrition out of food more easily. If you experience cuts on your lips, tongue, or inside of your mouth, then rinse your mouth with salt water regularly. Also, mention this to your doctor, because it could be a symptom of some other health condition as well.

After the occurrence of stroke or heart attack, it is possible that patient's head tend to tilt toward left forward or right forward direction. Patient may find it hard to keep the head straight up. Often, I thought this condition to be like a flowering plant which was wind blown for a few days, or got exposed to some heavy rains which made it to droop on one side. Somewhat similar seems to be the condition of a patient after experiencing a stroke or heart attack. Muscles and general weakness do not allow the patient to keep the head straight. In my opinion, this condition must be rectified just as soon as possible, because if unattended to, it may take a very long time to correct it.

To correct this **DROOPING HEAD CONDITION**, patient should lie down on the floor with as flat a position as the patient can manage. Patient or caregiver should try to see that patient's position on the floor is so relaxed and flat that most places of his back are touching the floor. Patient's neck should be straight while the back of the head is resting on the floor. Both hands should be on the sides of legs. There should not be any exertion on the neck. Now the patient should turn the head to the left in a slow motion. After a few moments, the patient should turn the head in slow motion to original position, that is, straight. After a few moments, the patient should turn the head in slow motion to the right. After a few moments, the patient should turn the head in slow motion back to the original position, that is, straight. To start with, this exercise should be carried out only in slow motion as many times as it is comfortable for the patient. The exercise should be continued until muscles are reformed and strengthened.

Similar to this exercise, there is another exercise that I would recommend. The second exercise is doing the same while standing straight against the wall, with back flushed with the wall. The back should be touching to the wall as many places as it is comfortably possible for the patient to do so. Both hands should be straight on the sides of legs. Patient should first turn the head to the left in slow motion, and after few moments in that left position, the head should be brought back to the its original position in a slow motion. Then, the patient should turn the head in slow motion to the right, and after a few moments the head should be brought back in slow motion to its original position. This exercise should be repeated several times every day, but only in slow motion.

Third exercise to correct the drooping head condition is while standing free of any support in an upright and straight position, the patient lowers the head in a slow motion so that the eyes can look at the feet. After a few moments, the patient lifts the head up in slow motion and brings it back to the original position. The original position is standing straight with head up so the eyes can look right in front. Similarly, patient should turn the head in slow motion to the right, and then to the left. These exercises must be carried out in controlled slow motion which will rebuild and strengthen the muscles surrounding the neck and upper back near the shoulders. Looking straight up will make the patient feel better, and eventually get better.

We did mention about the BITE ALIGNMENT, biting the food, biting the inside walls of the mouth, and the related difficulties. After the stroke lips do not seem to behave in the manner they used to do before the stroke. Smile is different. It is not a complete smile, because the FACIAL muscles are weak or lifeless. There are exercises which can help the patient to recoup the muscle strength of the mouth, lips, cheeks, and general countenance. Expressions are important component of any communication. Stroke and heart disease patients lose such communicative expressions, and therefore render themselves to be misunderstood, or misinterpreted. I suggest the patient to visualize the childhood days when most children used to make faces either to tease, mimic, scare, humor, or surprise others. In all these facial make ups, there is some muscle twisting involved. Stroke patient should exercise, in privacy of course, the entire facial make up reproductions. Taking the tongue out as far as it is comfortably possible, opening the mouth wide open to its limits, stretching the smile as wide as comfortably possible, making a yawning position, mimicking animal faces, etc. will definitely help the patient to rebuild and strengthen the facial muscles, which will improve the expressions as well.

I used a very affective way to increase **BLOOD CIRCULATION** in and around head area. I found this method to be very simple, easy to use, and extremely beneficial in the process of recovery from stroke. Take a regular cotton towel, and hold it above your both hands. Now your hands are below the towel. Gently rub the sides of your temple, forehead, cheeks, chin, lips, sides of the neck, front of your neck, ears, all around your ears including just below the ear lobe, back of the neck including the pit formed by the spinal bone and the ridge of your head. While rubbing the towel, press and squeeze with your finger tips on each location, especially on and on the side of muscles. You are massaging, pressing, and squeezing the area around your head and neck with your hands and finger tips behind the towel. Your hands and finger tips are not touching your skin directly, but through the towel. Just massage every possible place on and around your head, including ears, just for a couple of minutes each and every day. You will enjoy doing it, and will be pleased with the positive and relaxing results. After this, you can expand this massage to the rest of your body.

You will love it and feel good at the same time. I strongly recommend that this daily massage should be carried out by you without anyone's help. You are the only person who knows where it hurts, where it is soothing, where you need to massage a bit more, and how much or how little pressure you want to give on a particular spot. Besides, each day, your need for the amount of pressure, specific spots, and the duration of massage may differ, and it will be the most practical and efficient to conduct this massage by yourself at your will and in your privacy. This massage will be great for the stroke and heart attack patients who require stimulation to every part of their body after the stroke and heart attack occurrence. Stroke and heart attacks cause stoppage of blood supply to various parts which need to be gently stroked and stimulated. Towel Massage on the neck, especially on both front sides of the neck, is very beneficial to you. The Internal

Carotid Artery and the External Carotid Artery are located in these areas of the neck. Internal Carotid Artery supplies blood to the brain, while the External Carotid Artery supplies blood to the scalp and face. I carry out this towel massage religiously every morning. If you choose to extend the areas of this towel massage to other parts your body then please do so, and you will never look back for making such a therapeutically healthful decision. Do not hesitate to continue the practice of towel massage even after you get healed, because it is healing as well as good for the longevity. This will also provide you with an opportunity each and every day to inspect your body which is highly recommended. Giving your self a massage on daily basis is a great exercise which affords various bones and muscle movements, coordination, some balance, focus, and is soothing and peaceful. Why not to spend a minute or two daily to give your self this super self therapeutic massage, and get better faster than you had envisioned.

I would recommend another easy method to massage yourself to increase and maintain blood circulation in your body. Take showers instead of taking a bath. Every time you take a shower you expose all your limbs and skin, one at a time, to the shower. Water coming out of the shower head must have some pressure to be effective. Shower with comfortable water temperature and adequate water pressure can prove to be very soothing and therapeutic for the stroke patient. Besides, taking a shower every morning allows the patient to look through most parts of the body, and keeps the body clean and hygienic. I used this method daily, and I learned that by pointing the shower on the knees, ankles, feet, shoulders, arms, and the inside of your hands proved to be a great relief from aches and pains from lack of blood circulation and possibly from arthritis. In fact, in the distant past, I relieved myself of pain from tennis elbow and tennis wrist quite many times by putting them under bearably hot water faucet. It was a laborious process but it worked each time, I was able to cure myself of muscle aches, arthritic pain in my bone joints, bruised and torned tendons without any medication. Yet there is another super massage therapy to increase the blood supply in your feet and that is when you are in the shower every morning. Generally, most of us take shower facing the shower head. This time, turn your back to the shower and let the shower pressure fall on you back. Take a small step forward. Rest your left hand on the wall for balance. Lift the right leg and bend backwards, and hold it with your right hand in such a way that the sole of the right foot faces the shower head and gets the water pressure on the center of the foot. Keep the bottom of the foot in that position for a minute or as long as you can comfortably do so. You can do the same thing with your left foot while resting your left hand on the wall for balance, and holding your left leg with your right arm so that the sole of your foot faces the shower head and gets the water pressure in the center of the foot. Although you will find it to be a little ticklish in the beginning, but you will know after just a minute how great this massage exercise turns out to be. It will massage the area which is seldom considered for massage, yet the blood circulation in that part can prove to be crucial to good health.

To give yourself a head massage, take a towel and cover your head with it. Now, squeeze your head gently with your finger tips from top of the towel. Shape of your hands should be like if you were holding a ball. Go all over your head squeezing and putting pressure with your finger tips. It will increase much needed blood circulation in the outer layer of your head. Daily massage of your head with your finger tips on your head, covered with a towel, will maintain blood supply, and will make you feel good and relaxed. Just one to two minutes daily head massage is a wonderful self therapy for getting better. Your daily routine to massage yourself will generate confidence, a sense of accomplishment, and will empower you to take control of your getting well sooner. In doing so, you are in charge of the managing process of getting well.

We all should remember that repair and maintenance corporations and shops to attend to repairs on your cars, TVs, home appliances, buildings, computers, etc. are in business to earn profits. Profits are the incentives for them to be in business. The same motivation works for engineers, accountants, lawyers, and doctors, etc. **Medical services are business enterprises, and are there to make profit**, and to maximize profits from each incident and each case. Just remember when you go to a service station just for an oil change, and you are advised to change the wipers, transmission oil, fan belt and muffler, break pads, etc. More times you visit auto workshops, more you will realize that just about every thing in your car needs to be repaired or replaced. They mean well because they want to see you drive your car in good condition, and in doing so, they want you to buy their services voluntarily, or at times involuntarily. They want to increase their business with every visitor they get in their workshop. Now, what would make the healthcare providers not do the same thing? After all, healthcare providers have highly qualified professionals, expensive facilities, high liability insurance, sophisticated machines, etc. Of course, they want a bigger chunk of money in your pocket. Who can blame them, and who should?

We live in a free enterprise system where goods and services are provided to the general public freely and competitively. Such free and competitive marketplace provides incentive to the entrepreneurs to be innovative, risk takers, and thereby create new jobs and wealth. This is the very same economic engine which generates and motivates people to develop new technology, conduct research to develop new and modern science to combat disease and heal patients, and the healthcare professionals involved in this economic system want to earn as much as they possibly can. No one can buck this.

The only thing the patient can do is to make use of this productive and helpful system, and participate in it, and control the management of the process of getting well. Since healthcare system is a bit more cumbersome for an average person to comprehend, the authority and the resultant choice falls in the hands of the medical community. Average stroke patient would not know what happened to him or her, or what is required to be done. It is not like having a common cold which can be cured with aspirin and some rest, which is also known to everybody, because it is so common. For complications of a stroke occurrence, one needs more sophisticated skills than curing a common cold. The medical professionals who are equipped and trained for this skill to handle the needs of a stroke patient, make all the decisions from diagnostic to prognostic range. Stroke patient's body, well being, and future depend upon these medical professionals.

Whatever happens in the general population will generally happen in any business community. From this community we pick law enforcement officers, accountants, lawyers, auto mechanics, politicians, etc., and this very same community generates a number of incidents like: crime, fraud, shootings, murders, etc. Additionally, we regularly experience incompetence, irresponsibility, carelessness, errors, etc. in all professions including medical profession. Any of these negative attributes could prove to be devastating for the patient and the non patient. These devastating occurrences are taking place on daily basis across the country. In this modern age we have statistics which show the percentages of such incidents. If the percentage of crime is declining in overall population, then the probability of getting a decent policeman, auto mechanic, lawyer, or a medical professional increases proportionately. On the other hand, if the incidence of fraud, murder, and other criminal activities are increasing in the general population, then the chances of finding a decent policeman, auto mechanic, lawyer, or a medical professional decreases. We should create another analogy and, that is, to see how many workers in a certain community, adequately know their jobs and duties that are being performed by them. We will be amazed how many people do not know how to do their jobs, either completely or correctly or entirely. Then the incidence of communication comes in to equation. There is another equally complicated aspect and, that is, communication between the doctor and the hospital/clinic staff members, doctor and the patient, doctor and the pharmacy, and the related interpretations. Make sure that all written materials are either typewritten or legibly handwritten when receiving from the doctor or the medical facility.

Because, stroke was never on the minds of the healthcare professionals, stroke patients were quite often **MISDIAGNOSED**. Stroke may result due to a variety of complications in the brain, and somehow they have been linked to other diseases. There are estimated 200,000 people die each year in the hospitals due to the medical errors, and the question arises how anyone can prevent this catastrophe. This statistics gets scary when we are talking about stroke patients who lose many essential faculties of brain and body to participate in question and answer scenario. Stroke patients, loved ones, and well wishers should make every effort to ask as many questions as come to mind. Also, doctor's diagnosis and prognosis must be in writing. Patients must receive in writing about what the doctor thinks about the patient's condition during each visit, and what needs to be done to heal the patient. It is quite possible that what the doctor tells the patient may be different from what the doctor ends up putting in the computer data base. If for some reasons, the doctor misdiagnosed the condition of the patient, then it is possible that the other doctors with the same health-care group may never change the erroneous diagnosis. It may be either to protect the doctor in the wrong, or to protect the healthcare group, or just carelessness. I experienced this first hand. During my first visit to my healthcare provider, a doctor noted down a complete report, but during the subsequent visits, no one had that record of my state of health condition. And this happened again a few times later. I do remember that different doctors were assigned to me, and who left the medical facility for one reason or another without leaving any records of my statements given to them previously. Therefore, I suggest that every patient should have something in writing, in original or a copy, which describes the health problems a patient is suffering from. In this way, the patient can show that written material to other doctors for a second and third opinion. Also, the patient can make other people aware of the doctor being visited, and some specifics of the health condition.

In the recent years, National Stroke Association has been established, which most definitely marks the important step in the recognition of stroke, Additionally, Brain Attack Coalition has been established, which is a group of organizations that promotes educating the professionals and the government officials about stroke. They have recommended establishing Primary Stroke Centers to treat about 700,000 Americans who experience stroke each year. About 35% of these stroke sufferers, each year, require more advanced facilities. These Comprehensive Stroke Centers will have additional staff dedicated to treating stroke, radiology suites, MRI, and operating rooms which will be staffed 24 hours a day. It is estimated that about 100 Comprehensive Centers will be needed across the country.

Very few stroke patients receive adequate stroke care. Researchers have logged that only about 4% of the stroke patients were given tPA, clot busting medication. tPA is the only Food and Drug Administration approved clot busting medication. Also, 75% of the patients do not arrive at the hospital within the 3 hour window after having a stroke. According to some medical professionals, tPA must be given to the patient within the first 3 hours from the beginning of stroke symptoms. Public knowledge, recognition of stroke symptoms, and action are needed to take the patient to the hospital right away are crucial for the patient's well being. Also, it has been logged by various researchers that most patients do not receive the preventive recommendations from the medical staff to prevent another stroke. There is a combination of factors that could improve the treatment and its outcome for the stroke patients. Recognizing the symptoms, patient's arrival at the hospital immediately within 3 hours, attention and care by qualified, sincere, and caring medical staff, right diagnosis and right prognosis, written advice to prevent another stroke, patient's complete compliance and cooperation, patient's or well wisher's active participation and management of stroke condition are important. Other side of the equation is that there is a shortage of qualified medical professionals in the USA, and this has been witnessed and experienced by so many. There is shortage of qualified staff members in every discipline of healthcare provision.

Researchers around the world have found that intense speech therapy given to stroke patients improve their ability to speak and understand language. Inability to speak and understand language is called **APHASIA** and, in this regard, a special therapy has been recommended by various professionals. This therapeutic training requires stroke patient to speak only and not use gestures. So the patient is forced to speak without the gestures. Also language games have proven to be of help in regaining speech and language understanding. Some scientists believe that when the patient is forced to speak without gestures and gets involved in language games, it causes the brain to move the language ability to another area of brain which did not get effected by the stroke occurrence. Other researchers are finding ways to accurately predict stroke by various indicators like: blood pressure, cholesterol count, life style, level of stress, family history, etc.

National Stroke Association (NSA) has been quite active in promoting awareness of stroke condition as well as its treatment. NSA is a part of Brain Attack Coalition who is educating medical professionals and the government about Stroke. They propose the identification of primary stroke centers for the regular stroke patients, and the comprehensive stroke center with highly skilled professionals and equipment for the treatment of most challenging strokes. It is estimate that about 100 comprehensive stroke centers will be identified nationwide, soon.

As and when such aforementioned improvements take place, they will definitely contribute to the well being of stroke patients, which is after the fact. Obviously, a man or a woman has to experience a stroke occurrence before such advancements in medical help can benefit him or her. Such improvements in the provision of medical care will not be available to a normally healthy person. Hopefully, normally healthy people never have to avail the benefits of such medical advancements and the sophisticated medical facilities, just by keeping themselves healthy. Healthy people do not need to visit medical facilities except for regular check ups. If the proportionate number of healthy people increases, then a decline in medical industry and healthcare business may occur because the account base will be reduced. This creates a pleasant contradiction. On one hand the healthcare and medical industry provides a great number of jobs to the people, it creates wealth for our nation, and is a source of innovative advancements in physiological sciences, yet it thrives on the people who are not in good health. Therefore, unhealthy people provide healthy work environment and healthy revenues for the healthcare and medical industry.

Would the people want to remain unhealthy in large numbers so that enormous revenues and substantial job growth can occur in the healthcare and medical industry? Of course, the answer is no. The question is could the unhealthy people become healthy and get away from the healthcare and medical industrial services, except for periodic check ups? If the regular check ups are prudently instituted and astutely controlled, then it is likely that more people may come out as healthy people than currently do. People need to control their physical life, and actively participate in doing so. Often healthy people visit the doctor for a regular check up, and return with strange diagnosis which keeps them stressed for several months during which they end up making several trips to the clinic or hospital for tests and other evaluations. Eventually, some people do get out of this routine, while others don't succeed in doing so. How many times, various tests have proven wrong, mistakes have been made, wrong interpretations have been made, etc. cannot be estimated, and neither the devastating toll on healthy people. More people use the healthcare system; the more beneficial it is for the healthcare and medical industry. Conversely, if fewer people use the healthcare system, proportionately less profitable it becomes for the healthcare and medical industry. Resolution of such a controversial reality of our organized healthcare system will be among the greatest challenges of all times.

Obviously, it pays to be in good health, and this condition of good health can help all of us to avoid stroke or heart attack occurrence. Do take active participation in your mental and physical well being and in dealing with medical community in general. We should learn to live with the system we have created.

We take care of our health, we take pains to make a living, we save, we raise family, etc. only because we want to experience life. And we want to experience life for a very long time. Some of us do not wish to abandon this life for anything. We all have the will to live, and no one can deny that, under sane conditions. At the same time, as we want to experience life for a long time, we also want to enjoy it while skipping and hopping our way through life. Somehow, quite many of our enjoyments are surrounded by those elements which are generally not good for our health. Most of us are aware of such negative elements and the outcome of by participating in them. To broadly summarizing these elements, we come up with: excessive eating of unhealthy foods, alcoholic drinks, late nights, irregular life style, smoking, gambling, etc. Most of us do like to delve in these activities, and history shows that humans have enjoyed them for thousands of years. For the past several decades, various surveys have been conducted to determine what makes certain people live longer than the rest of their fellow humans. These surveys were exclusively focused on people who lived to beyond 100 years of age. Ironically, and to the dismay of many scientists, most of them drank alcohol, smoked heavily, ate all the rich foods they could comfortably consume, and lived an irregular life. Could it be possible that they had/have good genes? But their life style was or is basically fighting the longevity aspect of their genes. I feel surprised when I think of the oldest people in the world have been heavy smokers and drinkers all their lives.

Wanda Hamilton has compiled a list of a few oldest people. John McMorran died in Lakeland, Florida, at the age of 117 years. He smoked cigars, drank beer, and ate only greasy foods. His eyesight and hearing was in tact at the time of his death. In Milan, Italy, there are more than 35,000 who are between 85 and 95 years of age, and who are heavy users of cigars, alcohol, and fatty foods, and their pastime is to be in smoke filled bar. In addition to this age group, there are more than 600 Milanese who are above 100 and never gave up smoking cigars, eating fatty foods, and drinking alcohol. All of them live in Milan which is quite a polluted city of about 2 million people. There have been such people all around the world over period of time. There have been several celebrities who smoked and drank heavily, and at the fatty foods, and lived a relatively long life. Levi Celerio song writer, died at 91, the Queen Elizabeth, mother of present Queen

Elizabeth of The U.K., died at 101 years of age, Milton Berle, TV star who had been smoking since age 12, died at the age of 93 years. George Burns who smoked 20 cigars and drank unspecified martinis each day, died at the age of 100 years. Bill Wilder, a six time Oscar winner, died at age of 95 years. Isabella Gibson, still alive at 100 years, Wencelao Moreno of Ed Sullivan show, drank and smoked heavily, died at 103 years of age. Jeannie Calment smoked until her death at 122 years of age. Marie-Louise Meilleur of Canada smoked until her death at the age of 100 years. George Cook of U.K. died at 108 years of age. At her 100th birthday, Ivy Leighton claimed that smoking helped her to live up to that age. Mohammed Hussein of Lebenon, is believed to 135 years old. Narayan Chaudhari of Nepal is believed to be 141 years old.

Obviously, there is a lot of work cut out for biological researcher to accomplish. However, according to Nir Barzilai there are a few identifiable attributes to longevity. Most of the people who enjoy long life have high levels of good cholesterols (HDL). Also, the molecules that carry cholesterol in the blood stream in the body happen to be much larger in people with long life span. This means that cholesterol is transported out of the system much faster, and there is no room for accumulation of cholesterol in any part of the blood circulating system. Long lived people never happen to be in any kind of rush, and therefore do not mind leaving the tasks incomplete, to be completed another day. They are often late for the appointments. They are not in a rush, and also they do not want to beat the dead lines. These people are seldom involved in an argument, and never in the "must win" or "must achieve" mode. Their attitude is positive and well meaning toward themselves and others. Of course, they carry family genes of longevity which provides them the inherent opportunity to enjoy life much longer. Attitude has a lot to do with living a long life.

Do we really want to live a very long life while we are subjected to regimented routines of special diets, hospital visits, prescription drugs, fitness routine in gymnasium, and other electro-mechanical medical help, with hardly any time left to enjoy life? **Do the sick, needy, and old have to be**

the contributors and facilitators for the medical industry's escalating healthcare costs and burgeoning revenues? You can easily calculate how much money you have to spend on health insurance premiums, cost of medicines, cost of visit to your doctor or clinics, cost of testing procedures, cost of surgical procedures, time spent on attending to medical bills and related correspondence, cost and time spent on traveling to and from medical facilities, and the infections you get during your visits to the clinics and hospitals. The more times you visit medical facilities, the more chances are that you would be exposed to some kind of infection or virus. After so many visits, some people develop friendships with the staff of such medical facilities, and visiting them becomes a routine and a habit. What an expensive, unproductive, time consuming, and health hazardous routine it can become. There is an easy way to get out of this health hazardous and avoidable routine chore, and it is not expensive at all. Try to conduct as much business with your healthcare provider as it is possible over the phone. This is the second preference. The first preference should be to get to the status of good health when you never have to visit medical facilities, except for rare occasions of annual check ups. Once your visits are reduced to the minimum, your chances of getting a virus or an infection will also be reduced drastically. While at these facilities, avoid shaking hands, coming close to anyone, hugging, rubbing cheeks, etc. Wash your hands each time you return home from outside.

In olden times, kings or the local village leaders used to collect a portion of the farm produce in the form of tax. In those days, tax was primarily for the protection services that were provided by the kings and local village leaders. Do we see any similarity in today's world? In my opinion, the only difference is while in olden times there was only one entity collecting such taxes, today we face several of those. Medical profession in conjunction with healthcare happens to be one. Promote yourself by promoting your own interests. The first step should be to have complete control over your healthcare and well being affairs, and manage them yourself. Our healthcare system is commerce based system. We have to live within this system, and we should adapt ourselves to survive in it. We will best survive if we use them sparingly, and do not give them too much of our time and money. No one should be legally or contractually forced to visit a medical facility, or go through several tests, or to sit on a machine because the doctor wants you to do so. You do all these things only when you are convinced that it will be good for you. You have got to be the judge; it is your body, it is your precious time out of the remaining years of life, and it is your money that someone wants whether directly from your pocket or through the government's pocket. So many unnecessary tests, prescriptions and surgeries can be prevented just by being aware of the commercial environment of the system. To comply with this commercial system and to maximize our benefits from it, we should adopt an attitude which is best suited to our well being in a commercial way. **Only a commercial attitude will work successfully in a commercial environment.** The best scenario would be when the government launches national health plan which ensures all American men, women, and children of all national origins, races, colors, faiths and religion to have access to all of their health-care needs just by presenting one card. This will eliminate all paper work, payments, selection process of complex and difficult to understand health plans, unnecessary medication and surgeries, and the enormours expense related to it.

Prevention of stroke and heart disease is the best cure, because it saves life, suffering, huge medical bills, and lingering trauma. Besides once the body is damaged by the affects of stroke or heart disease, it is unlikely that it ever will be the same as before, and possibly some additional health problems may develop later. Hence, we must take care of the body we have and protect it from getting damaged in the first place by taking preventive measures. To prevent a stroke or heart disease, we require discipline and determination to stay healthy, and in the same vein we need to develop a positive attitude to stay healthy.

ATTITUDE governs several walks of our life. Positive attitude does bring positive results at least most of the times. If we have a happy attitude then we are happy and we make people around us to be happy. If we are happy we want to look good, and live longer. A positive attitude is necessary to live longer. Here are some positive measures we all can take to make our life a healthy one, and ultimately leading it to a lengthy and happy one.

CHAPTER VIII

CONCLUSIONS

SELF MANAGEMENT OF YOUR HEALTH

We all can start by selecting the right foods that are good for our body and avoiding or at least minimizing the intake of those which are not good for our health. You can read the nutritional values of most foods from the previous pages, and select your choice of vegetables, fruits, nuts, grains, beans, and other sources of protein. Make your own menu and recipes to suit your taste. You know your taste, and therefore you can improvise your menu each day to satisfy your needs. You have got to enjoy the foods you eat, and therefore menus suggested by others may not work for you. Also, it will be quite a chore to find all the ingredients in your kitchen cabinets. Who would store all those specialty food items and then assemble them for each meal? You may like to eat some meals outside from time to time, and you will be able to judge on your own what you like to eat and what is good for you. You will create a happy marriage between what is good for you and what you enjoy eating. Beans, lentils, peas, tofu, green vegetables, fruits, nuts, non fat yogurt, oat bran, fiber, fish containing omega 3, flax-seed oil, olive oil, dark chocolate, etc. are good for the body. Avoid or minimize the consumption of animal products as much as it is possible. Also, avoid consuming manufactured foods as much as it is possible for you. Minimize the consumption of sugar, and do take the vitamin supplement in conjunction and proportion to all other foods that you consume. If for some reason you do not consume sufficient amount of fiber containing foods, then do take a fiber tablet, daily. While always maintaining higher levels of HDL in your blood stream, have annual blood check ups to stay on top of your health issues.

Maintain a walking with optional light aerobic exercise schedule on daily basis, talk to as many people as you can, try to be outside of your living quarters as much as possible, live in a toxins and radiation free environment, avoid exposure to hazardous metals and chemicals, bring humor in to your life, and perceive everyone as a good person even though it may not be true.

Give yourself towel massage every day and cover all areas of your neck, face, head and other areas of your body, as I have suggested in previous pages. Give yourself shower massage and let the shower hit you just about every part of the body including the palm of your hands and the bottom of your feet. At least once a week if not twice a week, give yourself a rub with baby oil to maintain the skin moisture and its youth.

No matter how busy a schedule you may be maintaining on daily basis, give yourself plenty of time to wake up, get in to sitting position on the edge of your bed and stay in that position for a few minutes without fail each morning. You may like to occupy your mind with some aspirations, goals, prayers, thoughts of gratitude, or travel, food, friends, etc.

Eating onions, garlic, ginger, turmeric, cumin, cayenne pepper, cinnamon, lime or lemon, and vinegar, green or black tea, one or two glasses of red wine, red grape juice, etc. should become an integral part of your diet. Try to drink at least 10 glasses of water each day, preferably tap water or boiled tap water. Try to maintain a much higher ratio of liquids compared to solid foods in your body. Take in to account the fact that quite often we end up eating a snack when actually we are thirsty. To avoid unnecessary eating try a glass of water, first.

Cleanse your body from the outside by using soap and water during your shower each morning; cleanse your body from the inside by consuming sufficient amount of fiber containing foods and ample water thereby facilitating the bowel movement to be normal on daily basis. Cleanse your mind of anger, anxiety, grudges, animosities, revengeful feelings, etc. by giving yourself daily time to meditate, and through self hypnosis as outlined in previous pages of this book. You can design any kind of self hypnosis on your own, and if you decide to take this exercise to a more advanced stage then do read on it in books especially written on this subject. Creating your own therapies work the best because you know the exact reasons behind each of these emotions.

Eat small portions of nutritious food, complete all food intakes preferably 3 hours before going to bed, and create a routine of slowing down in your activities as your bedtime approaches. Try consuming the most nutritious portion of your daily intake of food by 2.00 PM and thereafter eat whatever else you wish to eat. Maintain the HDL (good cholesterol) levels high, and reduce the LDL levels by reducing the intake of animal products, fried foods, and foods which contain Trans fatty acids (AA). If you were an under weight baby at birth, then try to be extra careful by completely eliminating animal products from your diet. Strengthen the inner lining of arterial walls by reducing the quantity of LDL which will also reduce the quantity of oxidized LDL. Reduce blood sugar, and avoid malnutrition. Reduce inflammation in the body, which can cause pain messengers and white blood cells to rush to the scene to protect the injured or inflamed area.

Increase antioxidants in the body by eating all the fruits and vegetables you can eat. To a great degree I have been practicing this at least for the past 10 years, and it healed me from strokes and other health conditions. I admit to have violated my own rules several times and I got paid back without delay with bad health resulting in set backs.

It will be useful to know how LDL is handled in our body. A large quantity of LDL is absorbed by the intestines in our body. Then some LDL is picked up by the liver cell Receptors. Liver cells have between 2 to 8 receptors on their surface. More receptors will pick up more LDL which will be brought to the liver where from LDL will be sent out of the body via bile. The LDL which is not absorbed by the intestines along with the LDL not picked by the receptors of liver cells end up in the blood stream, and therefore getting identified as blood cholesterol. LDL in blood stream is bad and dangerous. When more LDL lands in the blood stream, it scores as high LDL cholesterol. Some people have more liver receptors and can eat a lot of food containing LDL and yet their cholesterol test will not show LDL to be high. If the liver cell receptors respond appropriately to the quantity of LDL at any given time, then all the LDL will be picked and processed by the liver and there will not be any LDL left in the blood stream. That is why so many people can eat as much fatty food as they wish, but with no ill effects. On the other hand there are people with either fewer liver cell receptors, or weak liver cell receptors in their body, who unless abstain from eating fatty foods can undoubtedly develop high LDL cholesterol in their blood stream. Here comes the subject of part played by the genes which is a hot topic of scientific research today. If the receptors are few or weak, then abstaining from all animal products should be exercised just as soon as possible.

Visit your doctor when it is absolutely necessary, and not before. Get most information over the phone, and try to avoid visiting clinics and hospitals. Also, if you have the slightest doubt or fear about the stress tests then do not hesitate to raise your questions or objections to obtain satisfying responses. Give your best try to keep your skin, intestines, blood, and mind clean, and you will end up enjoying a healthy life.

Try your best to avoid developing additional health problems on top of stroke or heart disease, and in this vein be extra careful about your health all the time. Wash your hands as many times as you can, and especially on returning home from outside. You receive professional assistance from the plumber for your plumbing needs in your house, auto workshop for your automobile, roofing contractor for the roof of your house, and medical professional for your health related issues. While all the professionals in your current life may have varied priorities, they all have somewhat similar business relationship with you. **Personal health is a major issue which requires immediate attention, but nevertheless it falls in to the category of commercial transactions, which happens to be the case with almost all activities we undertake in our life. So treat the healthcare providers exactly as you treat the auto workshops and plumbing contractors, which is what the environment of commerce demands.** Of course respect, courtesy, and acceptable protocol are valuable attributes to obtain the best out of every given situation. Your demand from the healthcare providers under commercial conditions are to receive the best diagnosis and prognosis in the shortest time possible with the most expeditious treatment and cure at the least possible cost. Unlike other services that are provided in the marketplace, healthcare is unique in the sense that error generated death cannot be replaced by new life or new body for the patient. Although all the demands posted by you may not get fulfilled, but if you maintain this line of thinking then you will end up accomplishing a lot more than you would otherwise. This attitude may reduce the probability of the incidence of medical error experienced by you.

Medical errors do get committed, and it will be difficult to determine the exact number of them, because even the fatal ones are difficult to prove. We have no choice but to live within the system until a better one is developed, and I hope that the new system is government sponsored and maintained, when various medical services providers become subcontractors of the government. This will transfer the major libel responsibilities from the medical community and the insurance companies to the government. Also, government will be more suited to regulate the pricing of healthcare than the private enterprise, especially in the healthcare business which involves the total population and national security, because the latter tend to merge and develop similar to monopolistic tendencies. Remember the old days when medical professionals used to make house calls and were more personal as compared to today when they seem to be doing a line job, just like on an assembly line. An average citizen who needs healthcare cannot be served adequately and justly under a system which has monopolistic tendencies under free enterprise economic environment. In the meantime, maintain good healthy habits, have a humorous, friendly and positive disposition, do make sure to minimize the occurrence of medical errors and undue infections and virus attacks by limiting your visits to the medical facilities to absolute minimum. You can only accomplish this by being in complete control of your healthcare.

Research in genetics has been going on for some time now, and each year there is a record of significant advancement in genes future role in the physiological healing process. It is estimated that within 20 years period medical science is expected to use specific genes to repair and heal specific portions of the body without any special medication or surgery. It may seem a miracle at this time, but it is expected that genes will be used to re grow certain body parts that have been inflicted by disease or rendered useless. Also, gene therapy may be able to stimulate growth of new blood vessels to and from the heart and making bypass surgery and many heart related surgeries obsolete. Until then and even after such advancement I suggest that healthy lifestyle and its self management should be religiously adopted.

Prem K. Bhandari (October 2006)

978-0-595-41870-1
0-595-41870-8